Notes on Obst

Please Return :

Liverpool MK/AD 2NU.

England.

NOTES ON NURSING SERIES

Notes on Gynaecological Nursing
William C. Fream

Notes on Medical Nursing
William C. Fream
Third edition

Notes on Surgical Nursing
William C. Fream
Second edition

Notes on Orthopaedic Nursing
Jane Webb

Notes on Obstetrics

William C. Fream
MB, BS, SRN, BTA Cert. (Hons), STD, FCNA
General Practitioner, Casterton, Victoria, Australia.
Formerly Principal Nurse Educator,
Ballarat Base Hospital, Victoria, Australia.

SECOND EDITION

CHURCHILL LIVINGSTONE
EDINBURGH LONDON MELBOURNE AND NEW YORK 1982

CHURCHILL LIVINGSTONE
Medical Division of Longman Group Limited

Distributed in the United States of America by Churchill
Livingstone Inc., 19 West 44th Street, New York, N.Y.
10036, and by associated companies, branches and
representatives throughout the world.

First edition 1977
Second edition 1982

ISBN 0 443 02707 2

British Library Cataloguing in Publication Data

Fream, William C.
  Notes on obstetrics.—2nd ed.—(Notes on
  nursing)
  1. Obstetrics
  I. Title   II. Series
  618.2   RG524

Library of Congress Catalog Card Number 81-70597

Printed in Singapore by
The Print House (Pte) Ltd.

Preface

The synoptic format for those needing to revise a large amount
of material in a short time has been found acceptable in most
disciplines. Judging by the success of *Notes on Surgical Nursing*
and *Notes on Medical Nursing* this is the case in the nursing
profession too. Hence it was decided to add Obstetrics to the
series.

Written primarily for student midwives it is hoped that
others—qualified midwives, medical students, paramedical
staff—may also find it useful.

1976   W. C. F.

Contents

1. Diagnosis of Pregnancy

Definition. State in which female body harbours one or more fertilized ova giving support, protection and nourishment until expulsion.

Changes in pregnancy

Profound alteration of hormone production causes changes in physiology. Though many of these changes suggest pregnancy, definite proof lacking until positive evidence of live fetus is gained e.g. fetal heart sounds, fetal parts felt, quickening.

Early changes
    Amenorrhoea
    Breast changes
    Morning sickness
    Weight gain
    Skin changes
    Bladder irritability
    Raised body temperature

Amenorrhoea. Missed period in sexually active female suggests pregnancy. Other causes in otherwise healthy woman are rare. Menstruation occurs 14 days after ovulation when production of progesterone from corpus luteum falls off. If production of progesterone continues or increases, endometrium is maintained and menstruation does not occur. Main reason for continuation is presence of fertilized ovum. After implantation trophoblast grows rapidly and produces progesterone and chorionic gonadotrophin which further consolidates endometrium thus preventing menstruation.

Breast changes. Week or 10 days after missed period woman may be aware of full feeling of breasts. May complain of hypersensitivity to pressure from clothing, friction from movements of arms, sharp pricking sensations—almost painful in intensity. At 6 to 8 weeks, usually after two missed periods, breasts noticeably bigger, covered with visible veins. At 10 to

12 weeks nipples have grown, areola darker and sebaceous glands in areola enlarge to become visible small lumps— Montgomery's tubercles. Darkening of areola may extend beyond its margins to form secondary areola.

Morning sickness. Nausea on first rising in morning a very common complaint. May be accompanied by actual vomiting. Two thirds of women free from vomiting or not greatly upset by it. A third more than mildly affected and about one in six of these are quite ill and need treatment (Page 33, hyperemesis gravidarum). Period of most intense nausea and vomiting coincides with time when circulating chorionic gonadotrophin is highest.

Weight gain. Early increase in weight occurs long before any appreciable increase in size of uterus or its contents. Due to fluid retention, a feature of increased oestrogen also seen in some women on contraceptive pill. Rarely exceeds 3 to 4 kg in first two months. Often attention is drawn to it by tightness of clothing. Major weight gain in pregnancy occurs after the 20th week.

Skin changes. Darkening. In brunettes especially, increased deposition of melanin in areola, mid-abdominal line (linea nigra), face—may be general or blotchy and irregular (chloasma).

Striae. Rapid stretching of skin of breasts, abdomen and thighs while cutaneous fibres are softened under influence of increased circulating oestrogen causes splitting of the dermis. Underlying vascular tissue give new striae a blue or purple colour. Old striae from previous pregnancy, or other causes have silvery or grey colour.

Bladder irritability. Renal blood flow and glomerular filtration increases during pregnancy but tubular reabsorption remains at pre-pregnant level. Net result is formation of greater quantities of urine which may contain larger amounts of urea, glucose and amino acids. Larger daily volume and more irritant nature of urine accounts for frequency in early pregnancy. Later uterus extends over the bladder and prevents it filling to full capacity. Cystitis occurs more readily during pregnancy and excessive frequency may result.

Raised body temperature. Basal body temperature raised about 0·5°C by increased circulating progesterone. Occurs in second half of menstrual cycle and continues during pregnancy.

Signs which may be present in early pregnancy

Hegar's sign. On bimanual examination during 6th to 10th week fundus felt as firm globular mass while lower segment is soft and easily compressed. Later entire uterus is occupied by growing mass and distinction between hard fundus and soft lower segment disappears.

Jacquemier's sign. Vascular congestion of vulva and vagina gives blueish or violaceous colour. Caused by high circulating oestrogens.

Osiander's sign. Increase in size of uterine arteries and greater volume of blood through them give distinct pulsation to palpation in lateral fornices.

Later signs and symptoms

Abdominal enlargement
Quickening
Fetal heart sounds
Fetal parts
Braxton Hicks contractions
Uterine souffle
Ballottement

Abdominal enlargement. At 12 weeks uterus just palpable above symphysis pubis. At 20 weeks fundus reaches umbilicus. At 36 weeks, in primigravid, fundus reaches xiphoid. In subsequent pregnancies fundus reaches xiphoid at 40 weeks. Dividing distance between symphysis and umbilicus into four gives approximate level at two weekly intervals. Dividing distance between umbilicus and xiphoid into four gives approximate height of fundus at four weekly intervals. Method is very approximate but coupled with regular weighings and girth measurements good evidence that pregnancy progressing normally.

Primigravid uterus reaches xiphoid at 36 weeks. Thereafter uterus sinks lower into pelvis due to slackening of pelvic floor and relaxation of lower uterine segment. Mother finds breathing easier and action of heart less noticeable. This is called lightening.

Quickening. Mother feels movements of the fetus. Occurs about 18th to 20th weeks for first time. First real proof to mother that her baby is alive. Very important psychologically.

Fetal heart sounds. Though heart one of first organs to form, its sounds not audible until 18 to 20 weeks. May then be heard with ear against abdomen or with stethoscope. Heard much earlier with Sonicaid or similar Doppler machine though these do not pick up actual heart sounds but rather pulsatile blood flow through arteries. Heard at 12 to 14 weeks in skilled hands.

Fetal parts. After 22nd week head, shoulders, curve of back and limbs felt with increasing ease.

Braxton-Hicks contractions. Uterus contracts about every 15 to 20 minutes. These contractions are painless. Can be felt after 16th week.

Uterine souffle. Swiftly flowing blood causes a murmur heard clearly with stethoscope if background noises eliminated. During pregnancy flow through uterine arteries and placenta sometimes heard as soft swishing or blowing sound synchronous with mother's pulse.

Ballottement. While fetus floats free in amnion possible to cause it to bounce gently between fundus and cervix by imparting to it a sharp tap with finger in posterior fornix. Before 16th week fetus is too small for this to be done. After 28th week it is too big and fills uterus too completely therefore will not ballott.

Pregnancy tests

Urine of pregnant women rich in female sex hormones. Test performed to discover presence of these hormones. Human chorionic gonadatrophin (HCG) occurs only in pregnancy (and in certain tumours, see page 47). Hence if proved HCG is present in urine of sexually active female who has missed period, pregnancy almost certain. HCG testing kits put out by many drug manufacturers under trade names. They supply suspension of red cells or latex particles coated with HCG and a solution containing antibody to HCG. When mixed together antibody causes red cells or particles to agglutinate. If antibody solution mixed with urine containing HCG, antibody will be used up. When mixture added to sensitised red cells there is no antibody remaining to cause agglutination and red cells or particles remain discrete. i.e. agglutination is inhibited. However if urine contains no HCG, antibody not used up and subsequent mixing with red cells or latex particles causes agglutination and test is negative.

Test using coated red cells takes about 2 hours and is 98 per cent accurate. Test using latex particles ready in 120 seconds and is about 95 per cent accurate. When other signs and symptoms suggest pregnancy but agglutination test is negative, test should be repeated two or three days later or a different type of test performed on another specimen of urine.

Ideally urine should be freshly passed into a clean container, not necessarily sterile, after cleansing vagina with plain water. Early morning specimen more likely to be concentrated than one collected later in day.

Older pregnancy tests also depended on presence of female sex hormones in urine and their effect on sexual organs of experimental animals—frog, toad, rabbit, rat. No longer used.

Serum levels of HCG can be determined if necessary but test is lengthy, delicate and expensive.

Ultrasound

Beam of ultra-high frequency sound waves directed into abdomen and reflected waves detected. Reflected waves altered by medium through which they pass and by type of reflecting surface. Transducers convert reflected waves to form picture on television screen or to expose a photographic film thus giving visual evidence of contents of abdomen. Surfaces between solid and liquid reflect particularly clearly and presence of amniotic sac easily determined as early as 6th week. System used later in pregnancy to determine fetal abnormalities, site of placenta, size of fetus and its position. Unlike X-rays no harm to fetus results and method can be used repeatedly. Main drawbacks, cost of equipment and shortage of skilled operators.

X-rays

From 16th week bone in fetal skeleton can be detected by X-ray but hard radiation may damage any tissues in certain stages of reproduction. May also damage ovaries of mother. Damage is cumulative hence decision to X-ray should be taken only when information is absolutely necessary and cannot be gained by any other method.

Pseudocyesis

False pregnancy. Intense desire to have baby and pre-occupation with thoughts of pregnancy and motherhood may cause hypothalamic activity to such an extent that production of gonadotrophins is greatly increased. Diagnosis of pregnancy may be supported by amenorrhoea, morning sickness, frequency, enlarged breasts and abdomen. However, uterus does not enlarge. Woman is usually in need of psychiatric care.

Evidence of previous pregnancies

May be difficult because many signs can result from other conditions—gaping introitus, abdominal striae, laxity of abdominal muscles—but usually these plus darkened areolae, scar from episiotomy and slit-like external os indicate previous pregnancy.

Estimation of date of confinement

Human gestation period usually 266 day from day of conception but as exact day of conception rarely known it is usually measured as 280 days from the day of start of last normal menstrual period. If usual menstrual cycle is shorter than 28 days, deduct number of days less than 28 from 280, if normal cycle greater than 28 days, add number of days in excess of 28 to 280 days. Even so, minority of births occur exactly 280 days from start of last normal menstrual period. Most occur within 10 days before or after the due date.

Naegele's rule. To date of start of last normal menstrual period add 7 days and 9 months for expected date of confinement; e.g. last normal period started 10th March expected date of confinement 17th December.

Quickening. Five months from date of quickening gives rough guide to date of confinement. Not very accurate in primigravidae because mother never having experienced quickening before is unsure of first instance.

Height of fundus. Palpation of height of fundus above symphysis traditional method of determining duration of pregnancy. Highly accurate in hands of skilled nurses, midwives and obstetricians. Also useful in detecting abnormalities if fundus is higher or lower than expected from other information—big or small for dates. Not easy to determine in obesity. (See page 3).

2. Normal Pregnancy

Ovulation

Half million potential ova present in each ovary at birth. Less than 500 ripe ova discharged during fertile period of life.

Growth of ovary, ripening of ova and production of oestrogens controlled by follicle stimulating hormone (FSH) released from anterior pituitary. FSH controlled by a releasing factor produced in hypothalamus (FSHRF). Both of these, FSHRF and FSH itself, inhibited by rising blood levels of oestrogen. Cyclical nature of FSHRF probably controlled by presence of XX chromosomes. Reason for onswitch at puberty unknown.

Ova develop in special structures, the Graafian follicles. Follicles consist of a mass of cells, theca cells, which produce oestrogens. Theca cells surround a fluid filled cavity in which the ovum develops atop a mound of cells. As blood level of FSH rises one follicle develops faster than rest. Development involves maturation of ovum and greater production of oestrogen.

Primitive ovum is primary oocyte with 46 chromosomes. Development causes meiosis or reduction division resulting in ovum with 23 chromosomes. Completion of maturation of chromosomes postponed until fertilization occurs.

Ovulation occurs when level of luteinising hormone (LH) produced by anterior part of pituitary gland suddenly increases. Production of LH influenced by a releasing factor (LHRF) from hypothalamus which is in turn influenced by blood levels of oestrogen. Sudden increase of LH causes rupture of follicle and release of ovum together with surrounding layer of jelly-like material, zona pellucida, and a mass of granulosa cells derived from Graafian follicle—corona radiata. Minute channels through zona pellucida allow nutriment made by corona radiata to enter ovum.

Ovulation occurs about half way through menstrual cycle. Time betwen ovulation and onset of next menstruation remarkably constant at 14 days unless fertilization occurs. Graafian follicle reorganised after ovulation. Forms corpus luteum. Progesterone produced.

Spermatogenesis

Spermatozoa produced continuously, not cyclicly, from onset of puberty. Same anterior pituitary hormone as in female-FSH, responsible. Production occurs inside seminiferous tubules of the testes. Primitive cells, spermatogonia, reproduce primary spermatocytes. Each primary spermatocyte undergoes meiosis and forms four spermatids each containing 23 chromosomes. Spermatids mature under influence of Sertoli cells present in seminiferous tubules. Stored in epididymis until ejaculation.

Testosterone produced by interstitial cells of Leydig between seminiferous tubules under influence of LH more appropriately in males called interstitial cell stimulating hormone (ICSH).

Other secretions, from seminal vesicles, prostate gland and Cowper's glands added to spermatozoa at time of ejaculation to make up total emission called semen.

Fertilization

Semen deposited around cervix. Spermatozoa pass through external os. After ovulation mucous plug in external os changes its nature. Its protein forms long, thread-like strands which act as a filter and hinder passage of deformed spermatozoa. Before ovulation mucus has quite different structure. Nature of mucus can be used to determine whether ovulation has occurred.

Spermatozoa pass through cavity of uterus, enter Fallopian tubes and reach ovum in distal end of tube. First spermatozoon to penetrate zona pellucida causes unknown reaction which prevents entry of any other spermatozoa. Entry of spermatozoon triggers completion of second maturation division of chromosomes in ovum. Fusion of male and female chromosomes occurs and zygote is formed.

Sex of zygote

All human cells contain 46 chromosome. All female cells contain one pair of X chromosomes. All male cells contain one X and one Y chromosome. During meiosis all ova receive a single X chromosome. Half spermatozoa receive an X chromosome and half receive a Y chromosome. At conception recombination of sex chromosomes occurs. If the spermatozoon contains X chromosome child is female. If it contains Y chromosome child is male.

Occasionally meiosis abnormal and ovum or spermatozoon contains no sex chromosomes or more than one. Fusion results in abnormal zygote (see page 141).

Cleavage

After fusion, zygote rapidly subdivides. Solid ball of cells, morula, within 2 days. Traverses Fallopian tube slowly aided by peristalsis, fluid flow and cilia. Reaches cavity of uterus after one week. Morula now a hollow ball or blastula. Outer layer of cells has special ability to invade endometrium. Small collection of cells within blastula, the embryonic plate, provides material for new individual.

Implantation

Seven to nine days after ovulation blastula embeds into endometrium. Outer layer of cells of blastula, the cytotrophoblast, proliferates to form a spreading mass of cellular material devoid of cell membranes, the syncytium.

Endometrium called decidua after implantation. That part underneath the embedded blastula is decidua basalis. This and syncytium later develops into the placenta. That part covering surface of blastula is decidua capsularis which grows and expands as embryo grows. That part lining rest of uterine cavity is decidua vera. About 12th week decidua capsularis makes contact with decidua vera and merge with each other.

Usually implantation occurs in fundus or cornua. Occasionally it occurs in tube—ectopic pregnancy (see page 41) or low in uterus impinging on os—placenta praevia (see page 38).

Implantation occurs only if endometrium is prepared. Monthly preparation occurs firstly under influence of oestrogen from Graafian follicles then, after ovulation, under influence of progesterone from corpus luteum. Oestrogen causes proliferation and thickening of endometrium—proliferative phase of menstrual cycle. Progesterone causes storage of nutriment especially glycogen—secretory phase. As soon as implantation is successful syncytium produces progesterone, oestrogen and human chorionic gonadotrophin (HCG). Latter hormone excreted in urine and forms basis of pregnancy test (see page 4). Corpus luteum persists and increases amount of progesterone circulating for 12 weeks.

Development of embryo

Terminology

Ovum. From conception to Day 21.

Embryo. From third to 11th week inclusive.

Fetus. From 12th week to birth.

Rough guide to expected length of fetus in centimetres is: Square age in months during first 5 months. Multiply age in months by five during last five months.

Useful for estimating fetal age of abortions.

Four weeks. Embryo 1 cm long. Complete in sac about size of grape. Covered in chorionic villi. No human resemblance. Yolk sac prominent. Eye spots present.

Eight weeks. 3 to 4 cm long. Wt. 4 g. Sac size of hen's egg. Obvious human appearance, but head as large as remainder and sharply flexed on thorax. Arms and legs present. Genitalia not differentiated. Chorion frondosum at one pole.

Twelve weeks. 9 cm long. Wt. 56 g. Placenta fully formed. Umbilical cord present. Fingers and toes present but not nails. Eyelids fused. Skin red and transparent.

Sixteen weeks. 16 cm long. Wt. 150 g. Sex differentiated. Lanugo appearing. Meconium present. Heart beat discernible. Fetal movements present.

Twenty weeks. 25 cm long. Wt. 280 g. Hair present on head and brows. Lanugo all over. Vernix in creases. Finger nails discernible.

Twenty-four weeks. 30 cm long. Wt. 650 g. Eyelids separated. Eye lashes present. Skin wrinkled and red.

Twenty-eight weeks. 35 cm long. Wt. 1000 g. Legally fetus is now viable, but less than 20 per cent survive if born.

Thirty-two weeks. 40 cm long. Wt. 1600 g. About 60 per cent survive.

Thirty-six weeks. 45 cm long. Wt. 2500 g. Lanugo almost all gone. Skin translucent and less red. About 94 per cent survival.

Forty weeks. 50 cm long. Wt. 3500 g. Skin without wrinkles.

Plentiful subcutaneous fat. Finger nails firm and projecting beyond finger tips.

Fetal circulation

Fetal lungs not working. Placenta is organ of respiration, excretion and nutrition. Considerable mixing of fetal arterial and venous blood because of four temporary structures:

Ductus venosus	Foramen ovale
Ductus arteriosus	Hypogastric arteries

Ductus venosus. Blood comes from placenta through umbilical vein which enters liver and joins portal vein. Ductus venosus also links it to inferior vena cava. At birth umbilical vein collapses. Remnant remains in falciform ligament of peritoneum. Ductus venosus becomes one of hepatic veins draining from liver into inferior vena cava.

Foramen ovale. Intra-atrial septum pierced by this so that bulk of blood entering right atrium from inferior vena cava is shunted immediately into left atrium, thus bypassing pulmonary circulation. At birth when lungs expand pressures alter in pulmonary circulation and flap valve of foramen ovale closes thus preventing diversion of blood.

Ductus arteriosus. Communicating tube between plumonary artery and arch of aorta. Blood from right ventricle flowing through plumonary artery is diverted into aorta instead of entering lungs. At birth expansion of the lung vessels encourages blood in pulmonary artery to continue on into the lungs and ductus arteriosus closes.

The hypogastric arteries. Branch off from internal iliac arteries and become umbilical arteries. When cord is cut these atrophy but remain as cord-like structure between peritoneum and anterior abdominal wall.

Fetal skull

At birth part of fetus appearing first is known as presenting part. Important to know what part is presenting as subsequent management of labour depends on it. 96 per cent present skull first. Pelvic examination imparts information regarding state of cervix, nature of presenting part and its position. Of those presenting by the skull 92 per cent have chin flexed on chest and emerge with face towards mother's sacrum. Other parts of skull which may present occasionally are face and brow.

In breech presentation buttocks, knee or foot comes first. In shoulder presentation fetus lies transversely and often needs Caesarean section. Careful palpation can forewarn of possible complications.

Cranium made up of five bones joined by areas of membrane. Membranous parts between bones are sutures. Larger areas front and back are fontanelles. Bones are two frontal forming forehead, two parietal forming sides of cranium and one occipital forming back. Suture between frontals is frontal suture. That between parietal bones across top of head is sagittal suture. Crossing sagittal suture at right angles anteriorly is coronal suture between frontal bones in front and parietal bones behind. Crossing posterior end of sagittal suture is lambdoid suture with parietal bones anterior to it and occipital bone posterior. Where

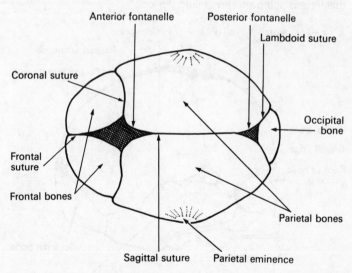

Fig. 2.1 Superior diagram to illustrate bones, sutures and fontanelles of the fetal skull.

the frontal, sagittal and coronal sutures cross is the anterior fontanelle wide and diamond shaped. Easily palpable. Where sagittal meets lambdoid is triangular space, posterior fontanelle. Less easily palpable.

Names of parts of skull are useful when describing position during stage 1 of labour. Sinciput extends from anterior fontanelle to chin (mentum) and is subdivided at root of nose (nasion) into brow and face. Vertex extends from anterior fontanelle (also called bregma) to posterior fontanelle. Occiput lies posterior to posterior fontanelle.

Fetal skull is not a sphere but an ovoid. Diameters of presenting part may be difficult to manoeuvre through birth canal. Most common presentation, well flexed head presenting vertex offers narrowest diameter to canal—suboccipito—bregmatic 9·5 cm. When slightly deflexed presentation is suboccipito-frontal 10·5 cm. When deflexed presentation is occipito-frontal 11·5 cm. When extended in brow presentation the diameter is mento-vertical 13·0 cm. When full extended in face presentation diameter is submento-bregmatic 9·5 cm.

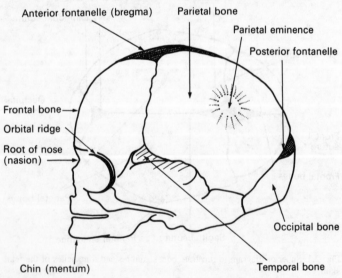

Fig. 2.2 Lateral diagram of fetal skull.

Sub-occipito bregmatic from below occiput at back of neck to the anterior fontanelle (bregma).

Sub-occipita frontal from below occiput at back of neck to the mid-point of the frontal suture.

Occipito-frontal from the external occipital protuberance to the root of the nose or nasion.

Menta-vertical from the point of the chin (mentum) to the centre of the vertex.

Sub-menta-bregmatic from the chin (mentum) to the anterior fontanelle (bregma).

Bi-parietal diameters from one parietal eminence to the other.

Bi-temporal diameter between the two extremities of the coronal sutures.

Other common terms describing position

The lie. Refers to relationship of long axis of fetus to mother, e.g. longitudinal lie when fetus and mother lie parallel as in vertex or breech presentation. Other lies are oblique and transverse.

The attitude. Refers to disposition of limbs. Usual fetal attitude is of flexion of all limbs and head.

The presentation. Refers to that part of fetus in lower uterine segment cephalic, breech or shoulder.

The position. Refers to the relationship of some fixed part of the fetus to some fixed part of the mother. Depends on presenting part. If vertex, occiput is reference point. If face, chin or mentum is reference point. If breech—sacrum. If shoulder—scapula. These are described in relation to mother's sacrum. Most common positions at onset of labour are with head transversely across sacrum and occiput on left or right side of sacrum. Shorthand descriptions are LOT and ROT. Less commonly occiput is directly anterior, OA, or directly posterior, OP. Occasionally occiput is halfway between transverse and anterior or posterior positions and lies to right or left of mother's sacrum. i.e. ROA or LOA when occiput is anterior and ROP or LOP when occiput is posterior.

Similar terminology used to describe position in othe presentations. e.g. 8 possibilities with face presentation are MP, LMP, LMT, LMA, MA, RMA, RMT, RMP.

Development of placenta

Syncytium penetrates deep into endometrium. Finger-like projections, the chorionic villi, radiate out in all directions. Each villus has a core of mesoblast cells which start to hollow out to form blood vessels and blood cells by 3rd week of pregnancy. Maternal capillaries erode when contacted by villi and maternal blood spills out to form lacunae from which nourishment is absorbed.

Penetration of villi goes no further than maternal arterioles. Just distal to furthermost penetration of villi special layer develops, fibrinous layer of Nitabusch. Ultimately cleavage of placenta occurs through this layer. On maternal side of layer of Nitabusch the arterioles are surrounded by myometrium which pinches them shut at birth.

Chorionic villi branch repeatedly. Smallest terminal twiglets end in capillary tufts separated from maternal blood only by a layer of trophoblastic cells. Although at first chorionic villi radiate in all directions, those growing into decidua basalis grow faster and deeper and larger lakes of blood form round them. These termed chorion frondosum. Those radiating towards decidua capsularis meet few capillaries and soon degenerate into layer termed chorion laeve.

Placenta fully formed by day 70. About 200 trunks of chorion frondosum enter from fetal side. Each together with its branches and terminal capillary tufts is termed a cotyledon. Sizes of cotyledons vary from 0·5 cm to 3·0 cm. About one quarter are truly functional. Cotyledons float in lake of maternal blood partly subdivided by irregular septa into inter-communicating compartments. Blood under high pressure enters compartments from spiral arterioles penetrating myometrium, cascades over cotyledons and leaves compartments through maternal veins. Flow rises from 300 ml per minute at 20 weeks to 600 ml per minute at term.

Veins on fetal side of placenta converge to form one umbilical vein carrying wholly fetal blood via cord to join portal vein and inferior vena cava via ductus venosus. Blood going to placenta is carried by two umbilical arteries—continuations of internal iliac arteries. Three vessels, two arteries and one vein, traverse cord embedded in jelly-like material, Wharton's jelly of fluid filled mesenchymal cells. Average length of cord 50 cm.

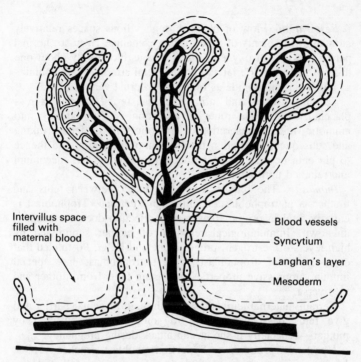

Fig. 2.3 Diagram of a chorionic villus greatly magnified.

Functions of placenta:

Nutrition
Respiration
Excretion
Immunity
Hormone production.

Nutrition. Small molecules pass readily through trophoblast by simple diffusion. All that the fetus needs is derived from mother's blood, water, electrolytes, amino acids, fatty acids, glucose, vitamins, minerals. Large molecules transported by active transport aided by enzymes and by pinocytosis, i.e. encirclement of solid particles and incorportion of them within the cell enclosed in vacuoles.

Respiration. Flow of blood through villous spaces relatively slow allowing plenty of time for gas exchange. Even so, normal partial pressure of oxygen in fetal venous blood only about one third of maternal arterial and normal fetal arterial blood contains as much carbon dioxide as found in maternal venous blood.

Excretion. Urea and uric acid transferred readily across placenta. Alternative route of excretion is from kidney into amniotic fluid. Reabsorption of amniotic fluid by fetal drinking and subsequent absorption from gut into circulation and thence to placenta occurs. Waste products in gut collect as meconium and retained until after birth.

Immunity. The only cell-to-cell contact between fetus and mother is at trophoblast/endometrium interface. Trophoblast is entirely fetal in origin. Reason why rejection does not occur is unknown. Immunological response of mother suppressed by high levels of oestrogen, progesterone and HCG. Postulated that outer layer of trophoblast, syncytiotrophoblast has special immunosuppressive properties protecting fetus from mother and vice versa.

Certain maternal antibodies pass through placental barrier and give fetus passive immunity to some diseases suffered by mother—especially if she has an attack during pregnancy.

Hormone production. Syncytiotrophoblast makes HCG. Level in urine peaks at 70–80th day of pregnancy, falls to lower level during rest of pregnancy and disappears entirely 7 to 10 days after birth. Functions of HCG: to maintain activity of corpus luteum until sufficient progesterone is made by placenta; to regulate oestrogen production; suppression of maternal immune reaction; other unknown fuctions.

Human placental lactogen (HPL) causes growth of secretory tissue in breasts.

Oestrogens made by trophoblast in gradually increasing amounts. They are in peak production at full term. Oestriol levels in maternal urine is an important measure of efficiency of placenta. Low levels indicate fetus getting insufficient nourishment, inadequate gas exchange and inefficient excretion of wastes and may indicate need for termination of pregnancy (page 94). Oestrogens enhance RNA production and protein synthesis. Many enzymes needed in placenta to bring about active transport of nutriment. Trophoblast manufactures these under oestrogen influence. Other functions of oestrogens—relaxation of cervix at term, increased size of myometrium, growth and mobility to nipples, laxity of symphysis pubis, relaxation of arteriolar walls in uterus ensuring greater blood supply to placental lacunae.

Progesterone also produced by syncytiotrophoblast. Converted to pregnanediol by liver. Level rises to peak at full term. Functions include inhibition of myometrial excitability and tone, aid in breast development, increase body temperature by about 0·5°C.

Probably other substances with hormone-like activity produced by placenta, one or more may be cause of increased activity of pituitary gland which makes greater amounts of throtrophin and ACTH during pregnancy.

Abnormalities of placenta

Normal placenta roughly circular, 20 cm diameter, 3 cm thick, with central cord.

1. Abnormalities of form

(a) Battledore: Cord leaves edge of placenta.

(b) Velamentous: Placental vessels traverse some distance in membranes before meeting to form cord.

(c) Succenturiate: One or more satellite masses of cotyledons occur separated from main placenta but joined to it by vessels.

(d) Circumvallate: Growth of trophoblast occurs laterally from edge of chorionic plate and membranes are folded enclosing a ring of decidua.

(e) Membranacea: Instead of definite placenta confined to one area a thin surface of placental tissue is spread widely over a wide area of decidua.

2. Abnormalities of penetration

(a) Accreta: Placenta penetrates through endometrium and meets myometrium.

(b) Increta: Placenta penetrates through into myometrium.

(c) Perceta: Placenta penetrates through myometrium to serous coat.

Such abnormalities prevent cleavage of placenta in 3rd stage and predispose to post partum haemorrhage and rupture of uterus

3. Abnormalities of site

(a) Praevia: Minor or type 1. Placenta dips down to lower uterine segment but does not encroach on os.

Praevia: Marginal or type 2. Edge of placenta reaches margin of internal os but does not cover it.

Praevia: Major or type 3. Placenta covers internal os (Page 38).

(b) Ectopic: Placenta implants outside cavity of uterus, usually in Fallopian tube but can be peritoneal or, rarely, attached to intestine.

Physiological changes due to pregnancy

Hormone levels. Oestrogens and progesterone levels rise throughout pregnancy. HCG reaches peak about 70th to 80th day and then falls to 25 to 30 iu per ml/serum by 20th week. Anterior pituitary hormones, ACTH and TSH also rise. ACTH causes increased levels of cortisone. TSH causes increased size of thyroid gland but higher levels of thyroxine not detected.

Cardiovascular system. Red cells, white cells and platelets increase in number throughout pregnancy. Total volume of circulating blood increases to about 5·5 to 6 l but as plasma volume expansion exceeds cellular volume expansion proportion of cells is less. Haemoglobin also falls but this is misleading. Although each individual red cell has less haemoglobin the total amount rises because there are many more RBCs.

Heart rate and stroke volume increase therefore cardiac output goes up by about 500 ml per minute. Hence, increased perfusion of all tissues affecting their functions. Diastolic blood pressure falls 5 to 10 mm. Systolic may do so too.

Urinary system. Increased blood flow causes higher glomerular filtration rate but tubular reabsorption remains the same. Hence products largely dependant on filtration for excretion are eliminated more readily, e.g. urea, and those depending on tubular reabsorption may occur in urine, e.g. glucose, amino acids, folic acid.

Dilatation of ureters and displacement of bladder in latter half of pregnancy favours urinary stasis and infection.

Water retention influenced by oestrogens. Extracellular fluid increased by 1000 ml or more. Probably intracellular fluid increased too. Dependent oedema common in last trimester. When persistent may indicate pre-eclampsia (Page 34).

Respiratory system. Breathing becomes deeper but not faster. Oxygen consumption increased by 20 per cent. Sensation of breathlessness occurs when uterus sufficiently large, but CO_2 partial pressure decreased.

Digestive system. Laxity of involuntary muscle throughout gut caused by progesterone. May lead to constipation, feeling of gastric fullness, oesophageal reflux (heartburn).

Nitrogenous foods, proteins, readily absorbed and nitrogen retained (positive nitrogen balance). Glucose absorption delayed and renal threshold lowered but blood levels not altered. Fats readily absorbed. Cholesterol level almost doubled in pregnancy. Minerals positively balanced—calcium, phosphate, potassium, sodium, chloride, magnesium and iron retained. Iodine excreted in urine and plasma binding of iodine increased hence free iodine and thyroxine reduced.

Skin. Increased pigmentation especially of face, areolae, linea nigra. Due to increased secretion of melanocyte stimulating hormone from pituitary gland.

Abdomen and thighs show striae due to thinning of fibrous and elastic tissue under influence of cortisone.

Sweat and sebaceous glands more active causing a greasiness of skin and hair.

Breasts. Pricking sensation and tenderness often earliest indication of pregnancy, even before missed period. By six weeks breasts obviously larger. Areola darker by 12th week. Nipples enlarge. Sebaceous glands enlarge (Montgomery's tubercles in areola). Veins dilate from 8th weeks. Clear fluid expressible from 12th week and colostrum from 16th week.

Uterus. Length of uterine muscle fibres increased × 15. Wt. of uterus increased tenfold to about 1 kg. Number and size of all blood vessels greatly increased. Early in pregnancy myometrium much thicker but becomes stretched and thin as time goes on. At term thickness is about 5 mm only.

Cervix firm and rubbery in first trimester. Soft, pliant and elongated until onset of labour. Gradually taken up and disappears during first stage as lower uterine segment drawn up over fetal head.

Vagina. Increase in size of vessels and blood flow give blue discolouration. Oestrogen causes laxity of collagen which allows great distension during birth. White discharge starts early in pregnancy due to oestrogen stimulation of cervical glands.

Weight gain. Total weight gained about 12 kg. 2·5 kg in first half and 9·5 in second half of pregnancy. About half this is fetus, placenta, amniotic fluid. Remainder is blood, extra fluid, breast, fat. If weight gain exceeds 500 g in four successive weeks in second half of pregnancy investigations for possible cause should be done.

Emotional changes. Depression and irritability common in first trimester. Placidity and contentment common later. Food fads and craving more traditional than real. Somewhat old fashioned.

3. Antenatal Care

Historical. In some respects antenatal care as old as pregnancy itself. All cultures take special care of pregnant women. In other respects antenatal care very modern. Only in this century special legal provision made for professional care, research into special problems, positive approach to pregnancy, early detection of complications, their prevention and treatment. Maternal mortality lowest in those countries where provision for antenatal care well established. Even so maternal mortality still occurs, between 20 and 30 per 100 000 confinements where high standard of care available. Estimated that perhaps 40 per cent of these are avoidable.

Common causes of death
    Pulmonary embolism
    Infection
    Haemorrhage
    Abortion
    Pre-eclampsia and eclampsia

Aims of antenatal care

1. Health of the mother. To establish general level of health at onset of pregnancy. To detect and treat maternal illness. To ensure adequate diet.

2. Health of the fetus. To detect pregnancy early. To ensure healthy environment for fetus by education regarding dangers of drugs, alcohol, smoking. To detect maternal and placental factors which could prevent proper maturation. To detect abnormalities of structure and function of fetus and discuss their implications with parents. To offer abortion in certain cases. To deliver a healthy, mature fetus by method which will harm it least.

3. Preparation for labour. To educate parents so that psychological barriers are removed. To investigate and ensure possibility of safe vaginal delivery or to make arrangements for alternatives at optimum time. To prepare mother physically.

4. Preparation for puerperium. To educate mother in her role. To ensure puerperium can be undertaken without undue physical or mental strain. To deal with special problems associated with single mother.

5. Preparation for post-natal period. To educate both parents in physical and psychological care of baby.

Parentcraft Education

An important part of antenatal care.

All mothers should be invited to attend parentcraft and relaxation classes. They are organised at most centres in hospital and in the community.

The aim is to inform mothers about the optimum behaviour during labour:

relaxation
respiration
thought control
muscle control.

Information is also given regarding re-adjustments during the puerperium, including care of her baby and her future role as a mother in a family unit. Family planning advice may also be included.

An increasing number of centres invite fathers to the parentcraft classes with their wives and some have special classes for fathers only. Some of the subjects discussed might include:

development of the fetus
physiological changes in pregnancy
his role as a father and husband
prevention of accidents in the home.

State Aid in U.K.

Full range of qualified personnel available to all pregnant women without charge—general practitioners, obstetricians, specialists in all fields, midwives and paramedical ancillaries.

Antenatal and postnatal clinics and services of specialist clinics upon referral.

Maternity hospitals, 'Flying Squad' ambulances, provision for home confinement.

Financial assistance—maternity allowance (£22.50 p.w.) from eleven weeks before expected date of delivery to seven weeks after, provided woman is not in paid employment. Maternity Grant (£25.00) for any child delivered after 28 weeks gestation alive or stillborn plus £25.00 for each additional child surviving more than 12 hours. Supplementary Allowances payable in cases of need.

Social workers can advise on special problems and enlighten parents of their entitlements under the law.

Special foods, milk and vitamins available at subsidized cost, or free under certain circumstances.

History

Full information required for maximum benefit from antenatal care.

Social
Family
General health
Previous obstetric history
This pregnancy

Social. Name. Address. Age. Marital status Occupation. Race. Husband's occupation. Income. Home circumstances—own house, flat, rent, other residents.

Much of this information obtained by Welfare Officer especially if mother reluctant to give it or if there is doubt of her ability to cope with the pregnancy.

Family. Any history in her family or father's of diabetes, mental illness, epilepsy, tuberculosis, syphilis, hypertension, twins. How many siblings and states of their health.

General health. Illnesses, at what age, any complications. Any operations. Any accidents, especially motor car accidents which involved pelvis. In particular any history of tuberculosis, diabetes, heart disease, kidney disease, poliomyelitis, rickets, hypertension. Fullest details of all treatment and investigations needed. Present status of ongoing illness established.

Previous obstetric history. Pregnancies. Live births. Stillbirths. Abortions. Duration of pregnancies. Complications. Dates of births, sex of offspring, weight and length at birth. Method of delivery of each. Any complications. Health of offspring—any deformities, any congenital illnesses. Present health status of each.

Health of mother following each delivery. Method of feeding.

This pregnancy. Date of onset of last normal menstrual period. Any nausea or vomiting, fullness of breasts. Any bleeding per vagina. Is pregnancy welcomed or resented? Has the patient been on oral contraceptives or had an intrauterine device?

Examination

Height. Weight. Age. Blood pressure. Careful examination of cardiovascular, respiratory and gastro-intestinal systems. Breast and nipple examination.

While performing physical examination any special features looked for and noted—any deformities, operation scars, evidance of needle marks on arms, state of skin—sepsis, eczema, psoriasis, pediculosis, general cleanliness. Oedema and its distribution. Varicose veins.

Samples of urine and blood taken. Urine examined for presence of sugar, acetone, blood, protein, bile.

Blood examined for haemoglobin, red and white cell counts. ABO and Rhesus groop, VDRL. Rubella antibodies and Australia antigen may be assessed under certain circumstances.

Pelvic examination (performed by doctor)

Speculum and bimanual on 1st visit to confirm pregnancy, to establish position of uterus, to obtain specimens for cytological examination, to diagnose vaginal infections, to ensure that vagina, os and uterus are normal.

In shy or apprehensive person it may be necessary to perform a one finger digital examination before a speculum examination, but most often the speculum examination is performed first. In this way cytological specimens are not contaminated with lubricant.

Cervical cytology

Patient lies in left lateral position with buttocks close to edge of table, lower leg straight, upper leg well flexed at hip and knee. Speculum inseted without lubricant. Good light essential. Cotton bud used to swab posterior fornix, wooden spatula to scrape external os, another cotton bud to obtain specimen from endocervix. All three specimens placed on one slide and slide immediately immersed in fixative solution.

Assessment of pelvic capacity

Most pelves can accommodate normal sized fetal head at term. Some estimate of pelvic adequacy can be obtained in all primigravidae and in those that had difficulty delivering a normal sized infant on previous occasions.

Measurements assessed readily are:

1. Diagonal conjugate.
2. Bispinous transverse diameter.
3. Intertuberischial diameter.
4. Sub-pubic angle.

Diagonal conjugate measured by inseting two fingers (taking all aseptic precautions) and measuring from point of contact of lower border of symphysis pubis on index finger to tip of middle finger which contacts sacral prominence. This distance, less 2 cm for thickness of pubis, is diagonal conjugate. Normal value about 12·5 cm. Often sacral prominence cannot be palpated without causing pain. This indicates an adequate inlet unless the examiners hands are unduly small.

Ischial spines palpated to feel if unduly prominent. Adequate space is 10·5 cm.

Intertuberischial diameter measured by placing knuckles of closed fist against perineum between tuberosities. Adequate diameter is 10 cm.

Sub-pubic angle should be rounded and and at least 85°.

Doubt regarding adequacy of pelvis resolved by radiography (see page 86).

Abdominal examination

1. Inspection
2. Palpation
3. Auscultation

Patient should lie comfortably on her back with head slightly raised and arms resting at sides. Bladder empty.

General shape and size of abdomen noted. Uterus rarely distends abdomen before sixteenth week. In later weeks fetal back usually lies to one side and makes that side more smoothly rounded. Uterus usually more elongated in primigravidae, more globular in multigravidae. Excessive abdominal size may be due to obesity, wrong dates, hydramnios, multiple pregnancy, fibroids.

Fetal movements may be visible after 18th week. Palpation extremely important. Can yield much information without risk to mother or fetus. Hands warm; patient exposed minimally; use pads of fingers, not tips; be methodical.

1st manoeuvre. With ulna border of left hand determine height of fundus above symphysis. Next determine what part of fetus occupies fundus. (This is not important before 28th week). With one hand on each side of fundus gently compress fundus. Fetal head is hard, can be moved independently of trunk, has an indentation at neck. Breech is less hard does not move independently of trunk and has no indentation.

2nd manoeuvre. Body of uterus palpated with palms of hands one on each side. Feel for fuller rounded curve of back on one side and less clearly defined and irregular shape of limbs on other side.

3rd manoeuvre. Facing patient's feet place fingers on each side of lower part of uterus just above symphysis. With gentle pressure determine if head is presenting. May be possible to ballotte head. When head well flexed and fixed in pelvis hand on same side as fetal back slips more deeply into pelvis than other hand. When head not fixed examining fingers tend to converge towards symphysis.

Pawlic's manoeuvre. Facing patient's head attempt to grip fetal head above mother's symphysis with right hand. Its mobility can be tested. This grip is not recommended as a routine measure. It can be painful.

Auscultation carried out with fetal stethoscope (funendoscope). Heart sounds may be heard as early as 16th week and should be heard by 20th week. After 28th week location of heart beat gives clues to lie and position of fetus. Most often beat heard best below umbilicus, indicating cephalic presentation, and on same side of mother's abdomen as fetal back indicating right or left occipito-anterior positions. In posterior positions heart sounds heard far out in flank. In breech presenation heart sounds heard commonly above umbilicus.

In multiple pregnancy maximum intensity of heart sound found in two (or more) places and gives additional clue to positions of twins.

Absence of heart sound may indicate fetal death, but alone is insufficient evidence. During labour heart sounds an important guide to fetal distress (page 88).

Subsequent visits

After 1st visit, mother seen monthly to 26th week, then fortnightly to 36th week, then weekly to term. At each visit urine tested for albumen, blood pressure recorded, questions asked regarding oedema—'Can you get your rings off?'—weight recorded, fundal height observed, fetal heart auscultated.

At 30 weeks blood taken for glucose tolerance test and 24 hour urine for oestriol. Often the general practitioner will share the antenatal care with the consultant obstetrician and a cooperation card is used for records.

Special care taken to ensure fetal well being. Greater risk to fetus if mother is: over 35, parity over 4, obese, short in stature—under 150 cm (5 ft), hypertensive, undernourished, a smoker or drug taker.

Fetal monitoring, especially in last trimester may include oestriol measurement, ultrasonography, X-ray, amniocentesis.

Advice given

Importance of adequate, varied, wholesome diet. Protein foods particularly important in last trimester. Iron and folic acid supplements given.

General health measures may need stressing—adequate rest, sleep, exercise, suitable garments, bowel habits, oral hygiene. Any questions mother may ask to be treated seriously and full explanations given. Often fears build up because of superstitions and ignorance.

Special exercises and relaxation clinics held regularly at most centres. All mothers should attend. Important lessons to be learned regarding optimum behaviour during labour—relaxation, respiration, thought control, muscle control.

Antenatal Fetal Diagnostic Tests

Recent advances in technology allow early diagnosis of fetal abnormality. Such tests not used routinely but only where there is reason to suspect abnormalities, e.g. in women over 37 years (incidence of Down's syndrome rises to 3 per cent); if a previous child had neural tube defect; metabolic defects featured in the family tree.

Tests: Ultrasonography—Amniocentesis for chromosome indentification and material for cell culture; alpha-feto protein levels; lecithin-sphyngomyelin ratio for test of lung maturity.

4. Abnormalities of Pregnancy

Multiple pregnancy

Definition. Two or more conceptions present simultaneously.

Types

1. Monozygotic (Uniovular, Identical). One ovum fertilized by one sperm. Early separation into two cell masses. One placenta. One chorion. Two amnions. Same sex. One twin usually develops more fully because of unequal distribution of blood. Occasionally cell mass fails to separate fully and twins are conjoined (Siamese). Occasionally one twin dies early in pregnancy and becomes shrivelled and flattened (fetus papyraceus).

2. Dizygotic (Binovular, Dissimilar). Two ova, fertilized by different sperms. Two placentae entirely separate functionally. Two chorions. Two amnions. May or may not be same sex.

Incidence

Twins 1 in 80 pregnancies. (Ratio of mono-to dizygotic 1·5.
Triplets 1 in 6400 pregnancies. Starts as dizygotic twins, but one ovum divides to become a pair of identical twins.

Quadruplets 1 in 512 000

Diagnosis. Suspicion roused by fundal height increasing beyond expected for dates and increasing rotundity. Palpation may reveal two heads or a multiplicity of limbs. Confirmed by radiography after 20th week or by ultrasonography at any time. Even so, 20 per cent of multiple pregnancies remain unsuspected until delivery.

Misdiagnosis common. Other conditions mistaken for twins: fibroid, ovarian cyst, hydramnios, retention of urine.

Certain diagnosis if two fetal heartbeats are heard by two people listening simultaneously one tapping out his count with his finger so that other listener can detect asynchrony of two beats.

Dangers of multiple pregnancy

Pre-eclampsia three times more common. Anaemia, macrocytic and megaloblastic because of increased demand for folic acid.

Premature labour because of increased bulk. Placenta praevia because of larger size of placenta. Post partum haemorrhage because of larger placental site.

Higher incidence of 'minor' ailments of pregnancy—morning sickness, varicose veins, swelling of ankles, tiredness, backache.

Twins often born before full term, often smaller than singleton (though combined weight more than singleton). Hence higher incidence of ailments affecting premature babes—respiratory distress syndrome, hypoglycaemia, hypothermia, cerebral injury, atelectasis, jaundice, infections.

Care during pregnancy
Mother should have more rest especially after week 30. Wise to admit to hospital to ensure rest between 32nd and 36th week. Diet should contain extra proteins, and be supplemented with iron, folic acid, calcium.

Mother should be seen weekly from time of diagnosis and sharp watch kept for signs of pre-eclampsia-proteinuria, hypertension, oedema.

Care during labour
Delivery made ideally with obstetrician, anaesthetist and paediatrician present. Good results with caudal anaesthetic, episiotomy, forceps delivery of 1st twin, rapid assurance of longitudinal lie of 2nd twin, oxytocin drip in readiness in case contractions do not resume soon after 1st delivery, and speedy completion of third stage followed by IV and IM oxytocin.

Common presentations
    Both cephalic 45 per cent.
    1st cephalic, 2nd breech 25 per cent.
    1st breech, 2nd cephalic 10 per cent.
    Both breech 10 per cent.
    Others: cephalic and transverse; breech and transverse; both
        transverse.

Complications of labour
Delay in delivery of 2nd twin leading to hypoxia due to shrinkage of placental site. Prevented by rupture of membranes and mother bearing down or commencement of oxytocic drip.

Transverse lie of 2nd twin. Corrected by podalic version and breech extraction.

Inter-twin transfusion due to wide vascular interconnection. Prevented by avoidance of holding delivered twin higher or lower than uterus until cord clamped.

Delivery of first placenta preceding 2nd twin with possibility of haemorrhage—2nd twin delivered as quickly as possible and oxytocic given at once.

Locked twins. Rare but dangerous. 1st twin usually breech 2nd cephalic and second head enters pelvis before 1st head. Treated by manually pushing 2nd head out of pelvis to allow completion of 1st twin. May need to sever head of 1st twin and push it out of way to allow birth of 2nd twin alive.

Hyperemesis

Definition. Accentuation of nausea and vomiting common in first trimester which, if untreated, may lead to dehydration, starvation, ketosis, with secondary, liver, kidney, heart and brain damage.

Vomiting in pregnancy covers complete spectrum from nothing more than occasional nausea on rising, through nausea and vomiting every morning in first trimester, through vomiting at any time of day to the severest form defined above which occurs in about 0·2 per cent of pregnancies.

Aetiology
Almost certainly due to altered hormonal balance. Increased oestrogen and progesterone causes nausea. HCG reaches very high levels in first trimester, coinciding with period when vomiting most severe, and then diminishes again.

Perhaps a high psychosomatic component just as some people suffer more readily from travel sickness.

Diagnosis
Careful history taken to eliminate other possible causes of vomiting—infection, dietary indiscretion, drugs.

Blood taken for full examination, urea and creatinine, electrolytes, pH., bicarbonate, pCO_2, Urine examined daily for acetone, protein and bile.

Treatment

Admit to hospital, correct fluid balance, electrolyte disturbance, and glucose depletion. Vitamin B complex needs urgent replacement to prevent cerebral damage and Wernicke's encephalopathy. Intravite B 2 ml IM daily. Vitamin B_6, pyridoxin (Pydox, Pyroxin) 25–100 mg daily orally or 50 mg IM.

Intravenous route is essential to bypass irritable gastro-intestinal tract. 3 to 4 litres of fluid daily:– 5 per cent glucose; normal saline in ratio 3:1. Usually 2 to 3 days sufficient. Reintroduce oral feeding when nausea absent for 24 hours. Give solid food—small meals at 2½ hours intervals. Fluids given midway between meals.

Sedation sometimes needed for 2 to 3 days. Chloral hydrate, phenobarbitone. Anti-nauseant drugs—promazine (Sparine) 50 mg 8 hourly, Debendox 10 mg t.d.s., meclozine (Anecolan) 25 mg b.d. Metochlopramide (Maxolon) 10 mg orally, IM or IV.

Pre-eclampsia: Eclampsia

Definition. Disease of pregnancy characterised by hypertension, oedema and proteinuria. Appears usually in last trimester.

Aetiology

Higher incidence in multiple pregnancy, primigravidae—especially in older women, in presence of diabetes, essential hypertension, the nephritides, hydatidiform mole, obesity, malnutrition.

Cause unknown. Many theories. In dogs placental ischaemia leads to state similar to pre-eclampsia. HCG levels higher and oestrogen and progesterone levels lower in pre-eclampsia. ACTH, cortisone and aldosterone levels increase in pregnancy and more so in pre-eclampsia. Much more common where there is mild to moderate dietary protein deficiency.

Signs and symptoms

Any two of hypertension, proteinuria, oedema, sufficient to diagnose pre-eclampsia. In mild cases, hypertension of 140/90 with a trace of proteinuria and no symptoms. In moderate cases, oedema of ankles persists and occurs not merely at end of busy day; hypertension more marked and proteinuria up to 500 mg per litre.

In severe cases generalised oedema—swollen fingers, puffy eyes; blood pressure raised continuously over 150/100; proteinuria greater than 1 g per litre. Symptoms include headache not relieved by overnight rest, blurring of vision, diplopia due to oedema of eye muscles, abdominal discomfort and tenderness over liver, vomiting, general feeling of illness.

Laboratory confirmation

No diagnostic test. Raised haematocrit due to haemoconcentration. Reduced plasma albumen. Raised plasma uric acid. Raised HCG. Reduced oestriol and progesterone.

Dangers

To mother—renal damage, liver damage, low fibrinogen coagulation failure, accidental haemorrhage, CVA.

To fetus—poor placental function, anoxia, dysmaturity. Higher perinatal mortality especially if eclampsia supervenes.

Prevention

Careful antenatal assessment with high index of suspicion. Prompt admission to hospital for closer assessment if weight gain excessive, any proteinuria, any hypertension over 140/90 after suitable rest, any persistent oedema. Ensure adequate protein and iron intake. Differentiate from essential hypertension, chronic renal disease, phaeochromocytoma.

Treatment

Mild cases, rest in bed on salt restricted diet. *Sedatives*: added in more severe cases, usually barbiturates. *Antihypertensive drugs*: reserpine, guanethidine, diazoxide IV if quick reduction of high pressure necessary. *Diuretics*: thiazides, e.g. chlorothiazide (Chlotride), frusemide, (Lasix), ethacrynic acid (Edecril), all used to reduce oedema by preventing reabsorption of sodium. Mannitol IV sometimes used.

Ultimately, cure for pre-eclampsia is to empty uterus. In severe cases not responding to treatment, induction of labour necessary (page 94). In less severe, cases aim is to keep pregnancy going until 36th week.

Most patients show at least some improvement on treatment. As long as improvement maintained keep pregnancy going. At first sign of deterioration, consider termination. Oestriol levels good guide to placental sufficiency. If urinary oestriol levels below 8 mg/24 hours at 30 weeks, 10 mg/24 hours at 35 weeks on two or more occasions, fetus is not maturing and therefore no point in continuing pregnancy.

Eclampsia is pre-eclampsia plus fits or convulsions, indistinguishable from epileptic fits. Mother most at risk, primigravidae, multiple pregnancy. Danger to fetus stops at delivery, but mother may fit post partum. Incidence of cerebral haemorrhage and accidental haemorrhage higher when fits occur.

Stages of fit

1. Aura. Unconsciousness, eyes rolling, muscle twitching of face, limbs. 10 to 20 seconds.

2. Tonus. General rigidity, head thrown back, breathing stopped, cyanosis develops. Up to 30 seconds.

3. Clonus. Alternating relaxation and contraction of muscles, maybe violent, tongue may be bitten badly, stertorous respirations, much frothy saliva. Up to 2 minutes.

4. Coma. Sleep state. Confused and amnesic if disturbed. Gradually passes off to normal consciousness. Occasionally merges into repeated fit.

Treatment

Aims: to stop the convulsion; to prevent recurrence; to reduce blood pressure; to reduce oedema; to deliver baby. Convulsion stopped by morphine sulphate 10 mg IV and thiopentone 200 to 500 mg IV. Magnesium sulphate solution combines anticonvulsant sedative and antihypertensive properties. 10 ml of 50 per cent solution given IM and 2 ml qqh. Depression of nervous system manifest by slowing of respiratory rate below 10 per minute and absence of knee jerks. Calcium gluconate given to offset such depression.

Hypertension combatted vigourously. Diazoxide (Hyperstat) 300 mg by fast IV injection very effective or Pentolinium tartrate (Ansolysin) 1 ml IM hourly until adequate fall achieved, or Reserpine (Serpasil) 2·5 mg IM 8 hourly.

Diuresis usually follows delivery but may be encouraged with frusemide (Lasix) 20 to 40 mg IV or mannitol IV.

Lytic cocktail, combination of (1) thiopentone, for rapid central sedation, (2) chlopromazine (Largactil) for prolonged sedation and lowering of temperature, (3) promethazine (Phenergan) for antihistamine, sedation and temperature regulation and (4) pethedine for analgesia. Mixture given IV in 10 per cent glucose. Rectal anaesthesia with Avertin preferred by some. Delivery of fetus. As soon as fits under control, possibility of vaginal delivery assessed. Amniotomy usually induces labour as uterus is irritable in pre-eclampsia and eclampsia.

If labour does not start within 12 hours Syntocinon drip started at 2 micro-units (1 ml) per minute (2 units per litre) gradually increasing to 4 micro-units per minute.

Caesarian section may be necessary, but avoided if possible because of high incidence of maternal mortality.

Hydramnios

Definition. Excessive amount of amniotic fluid. Normal value 500 to 1500 ml. 2000 ml detectable clinically.

Cause
Unknown. Source of amniotic fluid not clear. Possibly transudate from maternal membranes, plus secretion from amnion plus fetal urine.

Associated conditions
Diabetes mellitus, pre-eclampsia, multiple pregnancy. Fetal abnormalities, anencephaly, spina bifida, oesophageal atresia, hydrops fetalis, ectopia vesicae.

Signs and symptoms
May be no symptoms until last weeks of pregnancy when large uterus impedes movement of diaphragm causing dyspnoea and palpitations. Abdominal discomfort, oedema.

Signs include uterus 'large for dates' fetus ballotts easily, but heart sounds hard to hear and parts hard to palpate. Fluid thrill detected.

Possible consequences
Malpresentation. Premature labour. Prolapse of cord. Retained placenta more common. Associated malformations cause high fetal mortality.

Diagnosis
X-ray. Ultrasound.

Type
Chronic: Slow accumulation of excess fluid. Most common.

Acute: Sudden increase in amniotic fluid usually between 20 to 28 weeks. Painful abdomen, nausea and vomiting. May simulate accidental haemorrhage.

Treatment
Minor degress: Additional rest periods. Avoid strenuous exercise, support abdomen.

If fetal abnormality diagnosed, induced labour by rupture of membranes and syntocinon drip.

If no fetal abnormality, drain off excess fluid using lumbar puncture needle. Up to 500 ml slowly removed at a time.

Placenta praevia: (PP)

Definition. Placenta situated close to or overlying os, beside or before presenting part.

Causes
Late implantation. Uterine abnormality. Associated with fetal abnormalities and multiple pregnancy.

Incidence
One per cent of all pregnancies.

Complications
Antepartum haemorrhage, malpresentation, premature labour, prolapse of cord, anaemia, fetal death, fetal anoxia, postpartum haemorrhage.

Classification
Minor: Placenta encroaches on lower uterine segment but does not reach os.

Marginal: Placenta reaches os but does not overlie it.

Major: Placenta lies across os.

Signs and symptoms
Bleeding. Commonly after 30th week when lower uterine segment starting to form. Painless. Repeated. Variable quantity,

may be little or much. May not occur until onset of labour. May be precipitated by coitus.

High presenting part.

Diagnosis

Localization of placenta by:

1. Radiography. Soft tissues shadows and inter-tissue planes may indicate position of placenta.

2. Isotopic placentography. 200 micrograms of technetium 99^m in human serum albumen given IV. Concentration of radioactivity highest over most vascular areas. Placenta 100 per cent more vascular than any nearby structures.

3. Ultrasonography. Locates placenta accurately.

4. Examination under anaesthesia. If PP suspected digital examination carried out only in theatre with immediate facilities for Caesarean section. Hence not done at all until after 37th week.

Management

Admit to hospital. Cross match blood. If less than 37th week, confine patient to bed, sedate, transfuse. Maintain bed rest for a week after bleeding stops. Exclude incidental haemorrhage by speculum examination (but not digital). When diagnosis confirmed keep in hospital until 37th week.

If onset after 37th week diagnose degree of PP.

Minor degree: Allow vaginal delivery.

All others: Caesarean section.

Heroic measures justifiable only if mother's life at stake and no possibility of early hospitalization; e.g. pulling down a leg and applying traction to control haemorrhage.

Accidental haemorrhage: (Abruptio placentae)

Definition. Haemorrhage due to partial or complete separation of normally sited placenta.

Cause

Aetiology unknown. Contributory factors include hypertension, pre-eclampsia and eclampsia, multiparity, chronic nephritis, external version, trauma, traction from short cord, folic acid deficiency, Vitamin C deficiency, anaemia, sudden release of hydramnios. In most cases—no reason discovered.

Incidence
One in 70 pregnancies. About one-third of all antepartum haemorrhages.

Grades
Mild: Moderate: Severe: depending on size of separation.
   Mild: Up to one quarter of placental surface separated.
   Moderate: Up to two thirds.
   Severe: More than two thirds.
Older grading: concealed, revealed, mixed, less informative of severity. Used less nowadays. Almost all cases are of mixed variety.

Signs and symptoms
Mild. 60 per cent of cases. Blood loss less than 500 ml. Mother not clinically shocked, but usually alarmed. Needs reassurance, Fetus unaffected.

Moderate. Blood loss between 500 and 1500 ml. Shock, abdominal pain, uterine tenderness. Fetal heart rate above 160 or below 80. Fetal movements may be exaggerated at first and later stop. Fetal death common.

Severe. Blood loss over 2 litres, mostly retained. Shock severe, but often hypertension of associated pre-eclampsia masks true picture. Abdomen very painful and tender especially over uterus. Fetus usually dead.

Complications
Hypofibrinogenaemia, renal failure, pituitary necrosis. Fetal death. Fetal anoxia with consequent brain damage if it lives.

Treatment
Mild: Expectant. Admit to hospital. Exclude PP or other cause of haemorrhage. If at 37 W or more induce labour by amniotomy and oxytocin drip. If bleeding continues and fetal distress occurs perform Caesarean section. If less than 37 W and bleeding stops, discharge and observe carefully until term.

Moderate: Transfuse. Treat shock. Check for hypofibrino-genaemia—bleeding time greater than 10 mins, fibrin degradation products in serum. Be alert for this possibility if blood lost PV fails to clot. Monitor fetal heart. Consider immediate Caesarean section if distress occurs. Fifty per cent are in labour. If not, induce by amniotomy and oxytocin drip. Post partum give ergometrine and keep close watch on uterus which tends to relax readily.

Severe: Transfuse. Treat shock. Deliver fetus which is almost always dead. Usually spontaneous rapid delivery occurs. If not, induce or perform CS.

In this class blood may penetrate into or even through wall of uterus. Fibrinogen may be largely used up in clot formation thus causing bleeding tendency. Injection of 5 to 10 mg fibrinogen or 5 to 15 mg epsilon amino-caproic acid IV may be needed before Caesarean section performed.

Other causes of haemorrhage:

Incidental haemorrhage: Bleeding from cervix due to injury, inflammation, cancer, varices or polyp.

Idiopathic: Large proportion haemorrhages remain undiagnosed. Small haemorrhages without symptoms which are not repeated and pregnancy continues to normal delivery at full term.

Ectopic pregnancy

Definition. Zygote implants at some site other than endometrium.

Sites. 99 per cent in fallopian tube. Remainder in ovary or abdominal cavity. Of these implanting in tube 17 per cent occur in fimbria, 55 per cent in ampulla, 25 per cent in isthmus, 2 per cent in interstitial portion.

Causes
Unknown. Theories: delay in reaching tube with loss of zona pellucida and fertilization late after ovulation. Distortion of tube by previous salpingitis. Congenital abnormality of tube.

Termination
1. Tubal abortion. 65 per cent
2. Rupture into peritoneal cavity. 35 per cent
3. Secondary abdominal pregnancy. Rare.
In tubal abortion, conceptus may be absorbed completely; may pass into peritoneal cavity from fimbria and there be absorbed; may remain within tube and become surrounded by blood clot—tubal mole. In rupture of tube haemorrhage usually sudden

and severe often before pregnancy is suspected at about time of first missed period. Occasionally gradual bleeding. Occasionally bleed occurs into broad ligament.

Tubal abortion more common when implant in ampulla. Rupture more common from isthmus or interstitial implant.

Signs and symptoms

Amenorrhoea common—one or two missed periods. Lower abdominal pain accompanied by a faint at onset. Vaginal bleeding—scanty brown discharge, continues without clots. Usually mass palpable but vague.

Occasionally sudden massive devastating haemorrhage. Severe lower abdominal pain. Shock. Later pain and tenderness spreads to epigastrium with referred shoulder tip pain due to diaphragmatic irritation.

Diagnosis

Not difficult when severe, but subacute cases far from certain. Help from falling haemoglobin level, normal white cell count, slight pyrexia, positive pregnancy test, mass present, tender fornices especially on movement of cervix, laparoscopy, culdoscopy.

Differential diagnosis

Abortion, ovarian cyst, pelvic infection, appendicitis, ruptured corpus luteum, salpingitis.

Treatment

Laparotomy. Transfusion, preferably with cross matched blood. Plasma or rheomacrodex or Group O rhesus negative blood or blood collected from patient's own peritoneal cavity, filtered, may be used.

Examination under anaesthesia may precede laparotomy in doubtful cases. Often this precipitates haemorrhage so should never be undertaken unless facilities for immediate laparotomy are ready.

Salpingectomy usually performed as recurrence of ectopics extremely likely if conservative operation attempted.

Abortion

Definition. Termination of pregnancy before 28th week.

Causes
60 per cent defective ovum: chromosomal abnormalities, malformed fetus. 15 per cent defective implantation. 25 per cent maternal cause: abnormal uterus—retroversion, fibroids, congenital abnormality, incompetent os—environmental stress, high fever, Rh isoimmunisation, congestive cardiac failure.

Terminology
1. Threatened abortion. Bleeding during first 28 weeks taken to be threatened abortion until proved otherwise.
2. Inevitable abortion. Wide dilatation of os and placental separation make loss of conceptus inevitable.
3. Complete abortion. Fetus, placenta and decidua completely expelled.
4. Incomplete abortion. Some part of secundines still within uterus.
5. Missed abortion. Fetus dies and is retained.
6. Habitual abortion. Three or more successive pregnancies terminated by spontaneous abortion.
7. Therapeutic abortion. Pregnancy terminated before 28 weeks surgically or by drugs when the health of the mother would suffer by its continuation or because of substantial risk that the child would suffer such physical or mental abnormality as to be seriously handicapped.
8. Criminal abortion. Deliberately induced abortion by any means by any person for reasons other than legal reason by a qualified person.

Differential diagnosis
First trimester bleeding: Ectopic pregnancy, mole, cervical polyps, carcinoma, implantation haemorrhage, pyosalpinx, ovarian cyst, metropathia haemorrhagica.

Signs and symptoms
Threatened abortion: Bleeding which may be very heavy. Intermittent pains likened to 'small labour pains'. Os closed. This may settle down to normal pregnancy, may become inevitable abortion or a missed abortion.

Inevitable abortion: Bleeding, pain, os open. Fetus already dead. Proceeds to incomplete or complete abortion.

Missed abortion: Fetus dies but is not immediately extruded.

Other signs and symptoms of pregnancy diminish—breasts no longer swollen and tender, no morning sickness, uterus shrinks. End results: (1) complete absorption of fetus and membranes—common in first 12 weeks. (2) Formation of carneous mole—lobulated mass of laminated blood clot due to haemorrhages into choriodecidual space. (3) Macerated fetus—collapsed skull bones, liquified organs. (4) Spontaneous expulsion.

Incomplete abortion: Some part of conceptus retained. Bleeding continues and may be severe. Os open.

Treatment
Threatened abortion: rest in bed. Sedation, e.g. promazine 50 mg t.d.s. Cervical inspection to exclude other causes and ensure that blood is coming from cervix. Pregnancy test. If bleeding stops ambulate gradually. Inevitable abortion: If complete abortion occurs, rest and sedation for 24 hours. Then D & C. If incomplete abortion, uterus must be emptied before bleeding will stop. Give morphia 15 mg or Pethidine 100 mg. Operate in theatre under GA. Can be manual—'finger curettage', or sponge or ovum forceps—retained placenta grasped, forceps turned and removed. Repeated until no more retained product retrieved. Oxytocin 5 units given IV or ergometrine 0·5 mg;

or curettage—large sharp curette used gently preferable to blunt curette roughly.

Discharge may continue for ten days or so.

Habitual abortion: Occasionally (20 per cent) incompetent os present. Abortion may be prevented by insertion of suture to keep os closed. Submucous suture of strong non-absorbable material encircles cervix as high as possible. Left until danger of abortion or premature labour is over. Removed at 37 weeks or CS performed.

Other causes of habitual abortion sought—anaemia, uterine abnormality, fibroids—and corrected if possible.

Legal and criminal abortion: English Abortion Act 1967 gives clear guidance for legal abortion in United Kingdom. Two practitioners must agree that continuation would be detrimental to physical or mental health of mother, or any existing children of her family, or there is substantial risk that child would suffer from mental or physical abnormality to a degree sufficient to cause serious handicap. Operation must be performed in registered premises and notified to Chief Medical Officer of Ministry of Health.

In Australia, law less specific, but abortion performed when mother's life at risk by continuation. Common reasons, hypertension, chronic nephritis, cardiac disease, psychological reasons, rubella in first trimester. Any doctor may perform operation if he conscientiously believes it necessary. It need not be in special hospital and notification not required. However, doctors advised to seek second opinion especially if grounds are psychological and to operate only in reputable premises.

Abortion performed by person other than qualified medical practitioner, or by a doctor purely for social reasons, is illegal.

In some countries no reason is needed to abort, but in all it must be carried out by medical practitioner. In other countries all induced abortions are illegal.

Methods. First Trimester: Dilatation and Curettage. Carried out in proper theatre under GA. Cervix dilated with Hegar's dilators to size 12. Conceptus removed with sponge-holding forceps with twisting action to ensure no damage to uterus. Gentle curettage follows then digital examination. Ergometrine 0·5 mg given IM and cervix observed for bleeding.

Suction. Tubes up to 14 mm diameter with side hole inserted through dilated cervix. Suction at 600 grammes/cm^2 applied via ordinary theatre suction apparatus.

Second Trimester:
1. Hysterotomy similar to Caesarean Section.
2. Intra-amniotic injection of hypertonic saline.
3. Intra-amniotic infusion of prostaglandins.

In third trimester term 'abortion' not used, instead, 'induction of labour'.

Object usually to produce living baby under circumstances where continuation of pregnancy would be dangerous to mother, child or both. (See Chapter 8, page 94).

Dangers of induced abortion
1. Sepsis. More commonly after criminal abortion. Rare with modern antibiotics. Commonly organisms responsible *Clostridium welchii, Escherichia coli,* anaerobic streptococci, *Staphylococcus pyogenes, Streptococcus* group A.

2. Perforation of uterus. Instrumental. Into peritoneal cavity, bladder, rectum.

3. Embolism, from forcible lavage.

4. Red cell haemolysis from lavage solutions being forced into circulation leading to haemoglobinaemia and acute renal failure.

5. Haemorrhage.

Septic abortion

Definition. Infection of the uterus following abortion.

Incidence
Varies in different parts of world. Highest in primitive countries and where legal abortion is denied.

Causative organism
80 per cent endogenous anaerobic streptococci, staphylococci, *E. coli*, confined to decidua.

15 per cent spread to myometrium, adnexae or systemic. Clostridia and Gram negative organisms.

Signs and symptoms
Pyrexia, tachycardia, offensive vaginal discharge. Tenderness over uterus and in fornices. Leucocytosis over 15 000 per cubic millimetre.

Investigation
Vaginal swab for immediate smear examination. Culture and sensitivity.

Blood cultures. In severe infections—urea, electrolytes, blood gases, pH, fibrinogen studies.

Treatment
Pending sensitivity tests ampicillin 1 g 6-hourly IV and streptomycin 0·5 g IM twice daily. If gas gangrene suspected give anti gas gangrene serum.

D & C if bleeding persists. Transfuse if necessary. Gram negative septicaemia—severe form of post partum or post-abortal infection caused by endogenous organisms especially *E coli*. High mortality. Intense vasoconstriction of venules preventing venous return. Thrombosis of liver, pulmonary and renal vessels. Low cardiac output.

Diagnosis of Gram negative septicaemia
Low BP and low CVP in spite of adequate fluid replacement.
Pyrexia, leukocytosis. Occasionally leucopenia—grave sign.

Treatment
Blood and fluid replacement. High doses of mixed antibiotics,
e.g. benzyl penicillin 30 million units, 4 g ampicillin daily IV,
Gentamycin, Cephalosporin or other antibiotics known to be
effective against Gram negative organisms, may be used pending
sensitivity results.

Acidosis corrected by IV sodium bicarbonate. Chlorpromazine
50 mg 6-hourly reduces shock. Corticosteroids, e.g. Solucortef
500 mg/day for one week increases cellular permeability. Iso-
prenalin drip 1 microgram per minute dilates peripheral vessels.

Trophoblastic tumour

1. Hydatidiform mole. (Benign trophoblastic tumour).

Definition. Abnormal development of placenta. Multiple
cyst-like masses of distended villi. Name derived from resemblance to cysts of hydatid disease. Blood vessels scanty or absent.

Cause
Unknown.

Signs and symptoms
Vaginal bleeding which persists. Vomiting. Uterus usually big
for dates. Hypertension. Oedema. No fetal parts felt. No fetal
heart beat. HCG remains elevated beyond usual time for it to
decline. Ultrasound fails to detect fetus.

Differential diagnosis
Mistaken dates: Multiple pregnancy: Hydramnios: Fibroids.

Treatment
Aid expulsion by digital evacuation. Delay curettage for few
days because myometrium is thin and vascular.
If patient over 35: Hysterectomy.

After care
Weekly estimations of urinary HCG continued for six weeks and
thereafter at 12 weeks 6 months and 12 months. If raised after 6
weeks, D and C repeated. Choriocarcinoma suspected.

2. Malignant trophoblastic tumour

Definition. Invasion of uterus, with or without secondary spread to other organs, notably lungs and vagina, by trophoblastic tissue.

Types
1. Confined to uterus: (Chorio-adenoma destruens). Death, if untreated, from perforation and haemorrhage; 2. Chorion carcinoma. (Chorionepithelioma).

Widespread, rapidly growing metastases. Absence of immunological response allows unhindered spread.

Prophylaxis
Weekly examination following delivery of mole to observe normal regression of uterus. Examination of vagina for signs of invasion. Estimation of HCG which should diminish and disappear within 21 days. Chest X-ray especially if haemoptysis occurs.

Signs and symptoms
Foul smelling vaginal discharge. Vaginal bleeding. Enlargement of uterus. Anaemia. Loss of weight. Secondary deposits cause signs and symptoms by interference with function of organs concerned; lungs—dyspnoea, haemoptysis, haemothorax; liver—hepatomegaly, jaundice, alteration of liver function tests; brain—headache, CVA, coma.

Treatment
Methotrexate 10 to 15 mg orally for 5 days. Repeated twice if HCG levels do not fall. May be given IV over 2 to 3 days. Side effects—stomatitis, diarrhoea and vomiting, intestinal ulceration, aplastic anaemia, alopecia. Treatment administered as inpatient under strict laboratory monitoring of white cell count and platelet levels.

Other cytotoxics used, subsequently or concurrently—cyclophosphamide, 6-mercaptopurine, Actinomycin-D.
Follow-up at monthly intervals for 6 months then three monthly intervals for one year then annually. Pregnancy to be avoided for at least one year.

Hysterectomy used to be standard treatment and still advised if patient has had enough family.

Prolonged pregnancy

Definition. Prolongation of pregnancy beyond 294 days from first day of last normal menstrual period.

Associated conditions
Hydrocephalus. Anencephaly. Malpresentation. Contracted pelvis.

Results
Difficult labour because of increased size of fetus, diminished quantity of amniotic fluid. Increasing danger of fetal hypoxia due to diminishing efficiency of placenta.

Differential diagnosis
Wrong dates. Long menstrual cycle. Fetal death.

Diagnosis
X-ray to determine state of ossification helpful.

Management
Induction of labour at 42 weeks. Careful monitoring of fetal heart rate. Fetal scalp capillary pH. Preparation made for forceps delivery or CS if necessary.

Fetal death-in-utero

Incidence
One pregnancy in 200.

Causes
Placental failure, e.g. following abruptio, P.P. Cord entanglement. Cord knotting. Gross fetal abnormalities especially cardiac.

Signs
Cessation of fetal movement. Cessation of fetal heart beat. Cessation of uterine enlargement. Failure to gain weight. Regression of breasts. Pregnancy test may become negative. X-ray may show overlapping of skull bones (Spalding's sign), or gas shadow in heart or aorta.

Palpation of fetal scalp per vaginam reveals 'bag of bones' sensation.

Management
Majority expel dead fetus within 2 to 3 weeks. Occasionally placenta continues to produce progesterone which suppresses oxytocin secretion and uterus fails to contract adequately. Induction of labour with high dose oxytocin drip successful.

Checks of fibrinogen levels and clotting time continued until after delivery to diagnose early hypofibrinogenaemia.

5. Diseases which may complicate Pregnancy

Cardiac disease

Grading of severity of cardiac disease:

Grade 1: No disability. Lesion noted on physical examination or special tests.

Grade 2: Breathlessness on moderate exertion. Activity slightly limited because of dyspnoea, occasional angina, fatigue.

Grade 3: Breathlessness on slight exertion. No activity can be sustained. Comfortable only at complete rest.

Grade 4: Dyspnoea at rest. Congestive failure present. Angina common.

Cause. Rheumatic heart disease—mitral or aortic stenosis and regurgitation. Congenital heart lesions. Thyrotoxicosis. Occasionally cardiomyopathy. Anaemia. Hypertension

Effect of pregnancy

Depends on cardiac reserve and degree of compensation. Previous episodes of failure, cardiomegaly, pulmonary involvement, presence of fibrillation—poorer prognosis.

Well managed case should not suffer further cardiac deterioration. Management in association with cardiologist.

Patient's full cooperation essential.

Diagnose and treat promptly—anaemia, respiratory infections. Regulate weight. Arrange life with appropriate exercise, rest, sleep, diet. Admit to hospital if any signs of failure—oedema, pulmonary venous congestion, increasing dyspnoea. Termination of pregnancy for patients in grade 4 unless pressing need for family.

Failure treated vigorously—rest, diuretics, digitalis, oxygen, assisted respiration, bronchodilators, fluid and salt restriction initially, physiotherapy.

Valvotomy not contra-indicated by pregnancy. Best results between 16 and 20 weeks. Delivery performed with patient sitting up, using pudendal or caudal block and forceps. CS not considered unless there are other indications for it.

Hypertension

Definition. Blood pressure of more than 140 systolic and 90 diastolic occurring before 20 weeks.

Grades
Mild: 140/90 to 150/90; Moderate: 150/90 to 160/100;
Severe: Above 160/100.

Dangers
Small placenta and dysmature fetus because of spasm of arterioles. Higher incidence of pre-eclampsia, eclampsia, antepartum haemorrhage and abortion.

Symptoms
Usually none.

Diagnosis
Repeated measurements of blood pressure. Test urine for protein. Perform renal function tests. Exclude possible causes of hypertension—coarctation of aorta, renal artery stenosis, polycystic kidneys, collagen diseases.

Treatment
Lower blood pressure by adequate rest—physical and mental—in hospital if this is the only way it can be achieved. Reduction diet if over-weight. Restrict salt intake.

Medication. In mild and moderate hypertension safe sedation provided by phenobarbitone 60 to 90 mg daily, mild antihypertensive drug such as reserpine 0·25 mg daily. In severe cases more powerful antihypertensives used, e.g. Bethanidine starting at 60 mg daily and increasing gradually to effective level up to 4 g daily. Lasix needed if oedema occurs, 20 to 40 mg orally daily.

Progress of fetus monitored by urinary oestriol levels, growth of uterus, weight gain of mother. In mild and moderate hypertension satisfactory progress maintained to 38 weeks and labour induced then by amniotomy and oxytocin drip.

Hypertensive crisis
Sometimes seen in patients who have avoided antenatal care. Patient presents with headache, nausea, vomiting, epigastric

pain, confusion and apprehension. Danger of eclampsia immi-
nent. BP over 160/110.

Treatment. IV diazoxide (Hypostat) 300 mg in 20 ml normal
saline given fast—10 to 20 seconds. Set up drip. Give valium
40 mg in 500 ml 5 per cent dextrose 12 hourly to prevent
eclampsia. Observe BP hourly. Start fluid balance chart. Maintain urinary output over 60 ml per hour with oral lasix 20 mg.
Monitor serum electrolytes. Add potassium chloride to drip solution up to 6 mg per day as needed.

Anaemia

Most common complication of pregnancy.

Cause
Most commonly—iron deficiency. Stores depleted by (a) new
blood formation—red cell mass of mother increased during
pregnancy; (b) transfer of iron to fetus; (c) increased muscle
bulk.

If pregnancies repeated rapidly may be insufficient intake
between to restore body iron. Haemorrhage potent source of loss
of iron. In tropics—hookwork infestation major cause of
anaemia and consequent abortion, fetal mortality, maternal mortality.

Detection
Routine check of haemoglobin.

Signs and symptoms
Pallor, weakness, tiredness, dyspnoea on exertion, oedema,
tachycardia.

Prevention
Oral iron supplements throughout pregnancy. If diagnosed late
in pregnancy IM injection of Imferon or Jectofer. Safe if precautions taken. Injection deep into muscle. Oral iron stopped temporarily to ensure adequate circulating transferritin to bind free
iron. Not given if history of pyelonephritis. IV total dose infusion rapidly restores body content. Dose needed to restore
haemoglobin to 14·0 g per 100 ml blood calculated. Given in
normal saline. Antihistamine given orally before starting drip.

Initially drip run slowly for one hour and patient observed for reactions—hypotension, angioneurotic oedema, dyspnoea, pallor.

In very severe iron deficiency anaemia not recognised until very later in pregnancy transfusion of packed cells considered. Must be given slowly and over-transfusion guarded against with Lasix which can be added to the packed cells.

Other causes of anaemia
Folic acid deficiency because fetus absorbs much of mother's store. More common in developing countries. Almost always present in multiple pregnancy.

Diagnosis. Serum folate level below 3 ng/ml. White cells show hypersegmentation—more than 4 lobes per nucleus. In more severe cases red cells larger than normal and many oval in shape. Actual red cell depletion and lower haemoglobin are late manifestations but may occur very suddenly. Bone marrow shows megaloblasts.

Symptoms
As for other anaemias.

Treatment
Oral folic acid 5 to 10 mg daily.

Thalassaemia

Definition. Genetic defect of haemoglobin formation with excessive red cell destruction accentuated by stress such as pregnancy.

Diagnosis
Anaemia resistant to iron treatment. Circulating red cells reduced in number. Haemoglobin reduced. Cells vary in size and shape, often thin with outer rim and central region more dense—target cells.

Serum iron normal. Differential classification of haemoglobin shows excess HbA_2 and HbF. Nucleated red cells and reticulocytes increased.

Jaundice and splenomegaly occur in severe cases. In Australia 5 per cent of Italian population and 8 per cent of Greek have thalassaemia trait.

Treatment
Blood transfusion if anaemia suddenly becomes worse.

Sickle cell anaemia

Recessive hereditary disorder almost entirely confined to negros. Fragility of red blood cells and distortion of their shape. Sickle shape caused by elongation of faulty haemoglobin molecules when they become deoxygenated. Cells which have 'sickled' block small vessels in any part of the body. Haemolysis causes anaemia.

Signs and symptoms
Anaemia, jaundice, intermittent attacks of fever accompanied by pains in the arms, legs, abdomen.

Diagnosis
Reticulocyte count up to 15 to 20 per cent. Serum LDH raised. Bilirubin level elevated. Reduced red cell survival time. Sickling readily demonstrated by addition of 2 per cent sodium metabisulphide to drop of blood on microscope slide. Haemoglobin electrophoresis separates out abnormal Hb S.

Treatment
Transfusion to bring Hb to 12 to 14 g per cent during third trimester. Treat iron and folate deficiency vigorously. Observe for complications-gallstones from high bilirubin excretion, pyelonephritis, leg ulcers, pulmonary infarction. Prevent hypoxia which precipitates sickling especially when other conditions coexist e.g. heart disease, chronic pulmonary conditions, anaemia from other causes.

Diabetes mellitus

Definition.   Endocrine disorder with either too little insulin secreted or insulin made ineffective by anti-insulin globulins (antagonists).

Effects
Glucose unable to enter cells hence their fuel for metabolism obtained from fats. Excess fat breakdown causes ketones to accumulate.

Craving for carbohydrates causes obesity. High blood glucose causes urine to have high osmolarity and failure to reabsorb water against steep osmolar gradient causes excess urine output which in turn causes thirst and electrolyte disturbance.

Pruritus vulvae more common because organisms flourish in warm moist environment with high sugar content. During pregnancy insulin antagonist production increases. Antagonist substances cross placenta and affect fetal insulin/glucose metabolism in muscle causing large muscular baby.

Diabetes in mother may remain undiagnosed until pregnancy. Glucosuria common in pregnancy. Glucose tolerance test performed on those showing glucose repeatedly.

Management
Careful control of diabetes throughout pregnancy by special physician. Control problems arise in 3rd trimester because raised glomerular filtration makes urine testing an unreliable guide to glucose levels. Blood levels needed daily taken 2 hours after a meal and insulin or oral anti-diabetic drugs given to keep level down to 7 mmol/litre.

Patient admitted sometime after 28th week depending on quality of control. Efforts made to maintain pregnancy to 38 W unless pre-eclampsia, hydramnios or increasing ketosis intervene.

Delivery
Primigravidae—CS unless diabetes is mild and without complications. Multigravidae who have delivered vaginally previously may do so again after amniotomy and possibly oxytocin drip if labour does not ensue within 12 hours.

Urinary tract infections

UTI more common during pregnancy because lowered tone occurs in uterus due to high progesterone levels. Urinary stasis more likely. Organisms probably ascend from bladder. Commonly *E coli*.

Signs and symptoms
Urinary symptoms often lacking. Nausea, vomiting and anorexia common in early stages.

Usually, frequency, burning on micturition, occasionally suprapubic pain, occasionally loin or back pain. Pyrexia 38 to 39°C. Rigors. Urine contains pus cells.

Differential diagnosis
Vomiting of pregnancy, acute appendicitis, pre-eclampsia, accidental haemorrhage (concealed).

Treatment
Rest in bed. High fluid intake, if nausea and vomiting allows, otherwise IV fluids. Midstream specimen of urine collected before instituting chemotherapy. Septrin 2 tablets b d given pending sensitivity results then antibiotic of choice instituted.

Established renal disease

May have been caused by variety of diseases, e.g. repeated pyelonephritis, glomerulonephritis, collagen diseases, analgesic abuse, polycystic kidney, hypertension, tuberculosis.

Management
1. Establish degree of renal impairment—output, concentrating ability, creatinine clearance, urea clearance, serum creatinine and urea levels, 24 hour protein loss, presence of casts in urine.
2. If renal impairment very severe advise abortion. A rising serum creatinine very serious sign.
3. Examine patient at fortnightly intervals.
4. Admit at 28 weeks for complete bed rest.
5. Induce labour at 37 weeks.

Dangers
Abortion and perinatal deaths more common. Pre-eclampsia in one third of cases. Renal function further deteriorates after pregnancy.

Carcinoma

1. Cervical carcinoma
Cervical cytology performed on almost all pregnant women in developed countries. Abnormalities revealed in 0·5 per cent. Follow up smears and punch biopsy performed at colposcopy if possible. If invasive disease detected before 30 weeks—abortion or hysterotomy performed followed by hysterectomy and/or

radiotherapy. (Cone biopsy avoided because of high risk of abortion.)

After 30 weeks—allow pregnancy to continue to 36 weeks then CS followed by hysterectomy and/or radiotherapy.

2. Carcinoma of body of uterus
Almost never occurs during fertile period.

3. Carcinoma of breast
Occasionally occurs during pregnancy. Often grows rapidly under hormonal excess—oestrogen, progesterone, HCG.

Any lump examined by radiology or thermography or xerography if available, followed by biopsy and frozen section. Mastectomy and radiotherapy if carcinoma detected.

Uterine abnormalities

1. Myomata (Fibroids)

Not common in fertile age range. Are cause of infertility in older women. May cause abortion.

Signs
Irregular uterus depending on site and size. Often not detected.

Differrential diagnosis
Twins. Ectopic. Ovarian tumour or cyst. Salpingitis. Appendicitis.

Effects
Red degeneration causing localized area of tenderness. Often misdiagnosed and laparotomy performed for appendicitis.

Pressure symptoms if large, depending on structures compressed.

Management
Allow pregnancy to continue to full term. Allow vaginal delivery unless myoma lies in pelvis and obstructs delivery. CS if this occurs.

Myomectomy considered later if more family required. Not performed at CS because of danger of haemorrhage.

2. Congenital deformities

Normally two Mullerian ducts fuse to form one uterus, one cervix and one vagina. Failure of fusion wholly or in part can result in all degrees of double organs from two uteri, two cervices and two vaginae to normal one of each.

Commonly uterus cleft shallowly—arcuate uterus—or more deeply—bicornuate uterus. Occasionally septum persists in a single uterus and may extend to divide vagina. Occasionally septum divides vagina, but does not extend into uterus. Other variations rare.

Results in pregnancy
Abortion common. Abnormal lie, retained placenta, inadequate implantation causing placental insufficiency. Delayed second stage.

3. Uterine displacements

(a) Retroversion
Commonly corrects itself at 9 to 12 weeks. Occasionally procedes to incarceration.

Signs and symptoms. Pelvic pain. Backache. Constipation. Painful defaecation. Frequency, incontinence, acute retention. Uterus difficult to palpate abdominally.

Result. Abortion very common.

Treatment. Admit to hospital if spontaneous correction has not occurred by 12 weeks. Correction of position performed manually under general anaesthetic.

(b) Pendulous abdomen
More common in grand multiparity especially if mother is obese or if diastasis of recti muscles present. Back pain secondary to lordosis common. Delayed engagement in 1st stage of labour. Adequate support of abdomen by corsets essential.

(c) Prolapse of uterus
More common in older mothers. May persist until about 20 weeks when lifted back into introitus by growing upper segment. Treated by supportive ring pessary until this time.

Ovarian tumours and cysts

Ovarian tumours accompany one pregnancy in 2500. Two thirds, simple cysts, e.g. serous cystadenoma or pseudomucinous cystadenoma. One quarter teratomas (dermoid cysts). Other varieties individually rare, but make up one tenth.

Ovarian tumours rarely affect pregnancy. May obstruct delivery if incarcerated in pouch of Douglas. May cause pressure symptoms.

Complications of ovarian tumours may occur—torsion, infection, rupture, haemorrhage.

Signs and symptoms

Sudden onset of severe abdominal pain, tenderness, rapid soft pulse, falling blood pressure, pallor, weakness.

Differential diagnosis

Abruptio placentae, appendicitis, fibroid degeneration, urinary tract infection, intestinal obstruction.

Treatment

Complicated ovarian cyst needs urgent surgical removal. Uncomplicated cysts need elective removal depending on stage of pregnancy when discovered.

1st trimester: Leave until second trimester as many turn out to be corpus luteum cysts which regress spontaneously.

2nd trimester: Remove as soon as convenient.

3rd trimester: If in pouch of Douglas delivery by CS and remove cyst at same operation. If not, deliver per vaginam and remove cyst by laparotomy as soon as possible.

Danger times when torsion occurs most readily are 2nd trimester when ovary lifts out of pelvis and after delivery before uterus has shrunk back into pelvis.

Infections

2. Rubella

Rubella virus crosses placenta. In first trimester can adversely affect cell division causing deformities—heart lesions, deafness, blindness, microcephaly, mental retardation. Fetus fails to develop immunity and harbours virus for many months after birth. Virus continues to interfere causing encephalitis, hepatitis, anaemia and myocarditis.

Diagnosis

Serum of mother contains antibodies which cause positive result in haemaglutination inhibition test (HAI). Test is highly specific for rubella. Titre of antibody very high ten days after infection. A rising titre in two specimens of blood taken one week apart indicates recent infection.

Treatment
Positive evidence of rubella infection in first trimester good grounds for abortion. Spontaneous abortion occurs in many cases. Estimated that half such infections will abort or suffer major deformities. No specific treatment for rubella.

Prophylaxis
(1) Deliberately infect all girls with rubella virus while at school. (2) Active immunisation with Cendevax (live attenuated virus) if HAI test negative. If any danger of recipient becoming pregnant within two months of immunisation Cendevax not given because the virus is alive and may be as damaging to fetus as normal rubella virus. (3) Passive immunisation with human gamma globulin within five days of known contact with rubella. Value not proved.

2. Tuberculosis

Uncommon nowadays. Combined treatment with two antitubercular drugs very successful—streptomycin, iso-nicotinic acid hydrazide (INH), para-amino salycilic acid (PAS), rifampicin, ethambutol. Repeated sputum examinations made to determine patient is not infectious.

Examination of contacts essential: (a) to discover source of mother's infection; (b) to eliminate possibility of infection of infant after birth.

If mother infectious at time of birth babe removed until either mother made non-infectious or babe's immunity established with BCG inoculations. If separation not possible babe treated with INH and inoculated with INH-resistant BCG.

3. Herpes simplex and genital herpes

Probably caused by different viruses. May cross placenta and infect fetus. New born infants readily infected. Viraemia can occur with hepatomegaly, jaundice, thrombocytopenia fever, diarrhoea and vomiting.

4. Syphilis

Uncommon, but increasing.

Routine testing of all pregnant women—Wasserman reaction (WR), Venereal Diseases Research Laboratory Test (VDRL), Fluorescent Treponenial Antibody Test (FTA), Treponema Pallidum Immobilisation Test (TPI). If positive, mother given one mega unit procaine penicillin IM daily for 10 days.

Congenital syphilis results from intra-uterine infection by transplacental spread of untreated disease in mother. Abortion and intra-uterine death common.

5. Gonorrhoea

Greatest danger to fetus is during birth when infection of the eyes can occur. Ophthalmia neonatorum may cause blindness.

No satisfactory serological test to detect gonorrhoea. Urethral and cervical smears may reveal organism.

Treatment
Organism highly sensitive to penicillin, and many other antibiotics.

6. Viral hepatitis

Most common cause of jaundice in pregnancy. Reported by some authorities to be more severe during pregnancy. No apparent ill effects on fetus.

7. Other types of jaundice in pregnancy

1. Haemolytic
Bilirubin presented to liver for conjugation at a rate faster than liver cells can process it. Causes—any condition causing rapid breakdown of red cells—(a) infective, haemolytic streptococci, malaria, *Clostridium welchii*; (b) metabolic—thalassaemia, sickle cell anaemia; (c) drugs.

2. Cholestatic
Damage to liver cells prevents conjugation of bilirubin. Special form occurs in pregnancy due to heightened sensitivity to oestrogens and progesterone. Usually arises in 3rd trimester when

these are at maximum. Causes jaundice and pruritus. Clears after delivery.

Other more serious varieties are tetracycline induced fatty liver and idiopathic acute fatty liver. High mortality. Fortunately rare.

3. Obstructive
Mechanical obstruction to bile outflow. Not peculiar to pregnancy. Gallstones, cancer head of pancreas.

Difficult to establish cause of jaundice. Tests may help. Serum bilirubin, conjugated and unconjugated; urinary bilirubin and urobilinogen; liver function tests—serum proteins and protein electrophoresis, enzyme studies, SGT, LDH, gamma GT.

Other jaundice is multifactorial.

Local infections

1. Monilia (Candida albicans) (Vaginal thrush).
Yeast infection causing itching and profuse yellow discharge. Mucous membrane covered with membranous layer. If scraped off mucous membrane raw and bleeding. Swab shows branching yeast cells.

Treatment. Natamycin (Pimafucin) vaginal tabs 2 n. $\times$ 10, or longer in chronic infections.

Nystatin (Nilstat) vaginal cream or tablets applied b.i.d. $\times$ 14.

Econazole and miconazole preparation not to be used during pregnancy because significant amounts absorbed and effect on fetus not known.

2. Trichomoniasis
Common protozoal infection causing burning and itching. Discharge may be offensive and frothy.

Diagnosis. Fresh specimen mounted immediately on warm slide reveals highly mobile organisms moving about swiftly. Killed and stained large flagellated protozoa seen.

Treatment. Natamycin (Pimafucin) pessaries during first trimester. Metronidazole tablets (Flagyl) 200 mg tds for 10 days effective but not recommended until second half of pregnancy. Father given Flagyl also as trichomonads transmitted during coitus.

Rhesus factor

Absence of rhesus antigen from circulating red cells renders a person Rh negative. Such persons develop antibodies to Rh positive cells if they get into the body. Entry of Rh positive cells occurs by transfusion or by bearing a fetus which has Rh positive red cells. To stimulate production of antibody, Rh positive red cells must enter the mother's circulation in sufficient numbers. They may do so during child birth or during abortion.

Development of antibody to Rh positive cells has no deleterious effects on mother, unless she receives a blood transfusion of Rh positive blood. But antibody can cross placenta in subsequent pregnancies and haemolyse fetal red cells. Furthermore, subsequent pregnancies with Rh positive fetuses will act like booster shots and stimulate ever greater production of antibody.

Detection of Rh negativity
Blood of all pregnant women typed as part of routine antenatal care. If mother is Rh negative, grouping of father performed. If he is Rh negative too, all offspring will be Rh negative and no danger arises. If he is Rh positive and homozygous, all the children will be Rh positive. This does not mean that immunization of mother occurs in every case. Sufficient blood must pass from fetus to mother to stimulate antibody formation.

Prevention of antibody formation
If all rhesus positive cells entering mother's blood can be destroyed before they get an opportunity to stimulate antibody formation, no danger arises. This is done by giving mother an injection of human gamma globulin rich in antibody within 72 hours of birth of the baby (anti D gamma globulin).

Effect of iso-immunization on fetus
When antibody passes from mother to fetus Rh positive cells of fetus haemolysed. Resulting reduction of fetal red cells stimulates further haemopoiesis. Liver and spleen enlarge. Bone marrow becomes more active. Effect on fetus and newborn child depends on balance between destruction and production. Mild, moderate, severe.

Mild. (Haemolytic disease of newborn.) Haemoglobin between 14 and 18 g per cent.

Jaundice develops about 10 days after birth. Good prognosis.

Moderate. (Icterus gravis neonatorum.) Haemoglobin between 10 and 14 g per cent.

Jaundice at or soon after birth. Serum bilirubin level over 10 mg per cent and rising. Hepatosplenomegaly present.

Severe. (hydrops fetalis.) Severe anaemia and heart failure with oedema, ascites and hepatosplenomegaly cause death of fetus.

Care of immunized pregnancy

Presence of antibody (iso-agglutinins) sought at 28 weeks and 34 weeks. If present and especially if titre rising, amniocentesis performed. Presence of bilirubin in amniotic fluid causes absorption of transmitted light of wave length 450 millimicrons. The greater the absorption the greater the amount of bilirubin. Mild, moderate and severe haemolysis diagnosed. If repeated amniocentesis shows disease remaining mild, pregnancy allowed to continue to 38 weeks.

Moderate severity may be treated by intra-uterine fetal transfusion with Rh negative blood attempting to prolong pregnancy to 36 weeks. Induction of labour at 36 weeks, and exchange transfusion if serum bilirubin is rising fast or if over 20 mg per cent.

Severe cases usually die in utero. (See Chapter 10).

Smoking during pregnancy

Smoking now recognised to have profound effects on cardiovascular system which may hinder proper development of fetus. Low blood levels of carbon monoxide reduce oxygen carrying properties of red cells. Statistically, children born to mothers who smoked throughout pregnancy are less bright at school than those of non-smoking mothers.

Drug addiction

Many drugs are suspected of being teratogenic. Almost all drugs in sufficient quantity and in early stages of pregnancy produce abortions and deformed offspring in experimental animals. Drug addicted women unable to raise children to maximum potential.

Newborn infants of mothers addicted to heroin, and morphine show withdrawal symptoms and need special care. Whenever mother known to be addict, newborn transferred immediately to special unit. Withdrawal signs include tremor, hypersensitivity to noise and physical disturbance, convulsions, tachycardia, hypotension, vomiting. Symptomatic treatment may increase chances of survival. Death may follow failure to thrive or inter-current infections.

6. Normal Labour (Eutocia)

Definition. Spontaneous expulsion of fetus, at term, head first, without complications.

Causes

Multiple. Increasing sensitivity of myometrium. Increasing amounts of oxytocin from pituitary and possibly placenta. Greater amount of movement of fetus. Pressure on nerve endings in lower uterine segment. Oestrogen and progesterone levels at their highest at term.

Prodromal signs

Lightening. Two to three weeks before term uterus sinks lower into pelvis. Increased elasticity of fibrous tissues allows laxity of symphysis pubis, sagging of levatores ani muscles, stretching of lower uterine segment. With uterus sitting lower pressure on diaphragm is lessened. Breathing becomes easier. Heartburn lessens. Walking becomes tiresome. Frequency. Lower position of uterus prevents bladder filling to capacity.

Pains: False labour pains may occurs.

Onset of labour

Pains. Uterine contractions felt as a hardening of the uterus. True labour pains are regular; last about one minute; often accompanied by backache; disappear completely between contractions; may continue without much change in frequency or intensity for hours.

Show. Passage of mucoid plug from cervical canal. Amount of blood and colour very variable.

Dilatation of external os. As contractions procede lower uterine segment is pulled back over presenting part. Os must dilate fully before head will pass through.

Stages of labour

First stage. From onset of true pains to full dilatation of os. Duration varies. Primigravidae up to 14 hours. Multigravidae up to 7 hours. If duration greater than these times case reassessed, causes for delay sought and management re-planned.

Second stage. From full dilatation to complete expulsion of fetus. About one half to one hour.

Third stage. From birth to expulsion of placenta and membranes. Up to half an hour.

Changes during 1st stage

Myometrium. (Primary powers). Muscle fibres contract with each labour pain but fail to relax to their former length following each pain. They remain a little shorter each time—called retraction. Prior to onset of labour, contractions occur throughout pregnancy, Braxton-Hicks contractions, but these followed by relaxation without retraction.

Contraction with retraction makes uterus smaller and more closely fitting to fetus, packs fetus down into lower part and pulls lower uterine segment, which is thin and mainly fibrous, over presenting part. Division between upper muscular segment of uterus and lower fibrous segment is 'retraction ring'. May be markedly pronounced and easily palpable in obstructed labour when called 'Bandl's ring'.

At onset of labour cervix is thick, fleshy, soft, easily palpable, protruding into vagina. As retraction progresses and lower uterine segment is taken up, cervix is pulled against presenting part. If membranes intact presenting part is cushioned by forewaters. Size of os estimated in centimetres. May be used to subdivide first stage into latent and active phases. Latent phase until os is 2 cm wide, active phase from 2 cm to full dilatation.

Membranes bulge through dilating os and amniotic fluid cushions presenting part. Tight fit of fetal head in pelvis separates amniotic fluid into two compartments—that in front of head is the forewaters, and that following head around the body is the hindwaters. Contractions of uterus transmitted via hindwaters to exert even pressure over fetal body. Maximum expulsive effective when head is presenting part.

In breech and other presentations the fit is less exact and free communication between hind and forewaters persists. Contractions push more and more hindwaters into forewater compartment and expulsive force on fetus is less efficient.

Membranes may rupture at any time during pregnancy causing discharge of pale odourless fluid. Easily mistaken for urine.

Ideally membranes remain intact until os fully dilated. Earlier rupture indicates possible route of infection. If labour does not follow rupture a prophylactic course of antibiotic advisable. Loss of large amounts of amniotic fluid before onset of labour may allow moulding of uterus round fetus and make expulsion difficult and painful. Deliberate rupture of membranes is favoured method of inducing labour. (See page 94).

During 1st stage mother encouraged to relax and not 'bear down'. Ante-natal education now bears fruit.

Changes during 2nd stage

Uterus contracts more frequently and more forcibly. Pressure by fundus of uterus against breech constitutes fetal axis pressure. When os fully dilated secondary powers come into play. Voluntary contraction of abdominal muscles and diaphragm help fetus to traverse birth canal. Maximum effect if secondary and primary power combine; that is mother bears down during pains and relaxes between pains.

When head reaches pelvic floor vagina dilates, rectum is compressed, any faeces expelled, bladder lifts above symphysis pubis and perineum thins out and stretches.

With each contraction head projects a little further. Between contractions head may recede again. Crowning occurs when occipital prominence escapes under symphysis pubis and no longer recedes between contractions. Perineum then sweeps over face and head is born followed by anterior shoulder, posterior shoulder then rest of body.

Changes during 3rd stage

After expulsion of fetus uterus continues to contract. Placenta cleaves away at fibrinous plane of Nitabusch. Cleavage may occur at centre and then peel away to edges—Schultze method—or it may detach at one edge first and strip away progressively to opposite edge—Matthews Duncan method. Membranes strip off decidua aided by gentle traction and twisting on the placenta.

Mechanisms of labour

Definition. Movements undergone passively by the fetus as it is forced through the birth canal, knowledge of which makes management of labour more rational. Mechanisms vary with lie, presentation, attitude and position. Understanding of mechanisms demands knowledge of shape, size, boundaries of birth canal.

Birth canal

Roughly tubular bounded posteriorly by sacrum, coccyx and perineum, anteriorly by symphysis pubis, laterally by ischia, sacro-spinous ligaments and obturator ligaments and membranes.

Tube takes 90 degree turn parallel to anterior sacral surface—the curve of Carus.

Inlet to canal bounded by bone all round—sacral prominence and alae posteriorly, iliopectineal lines laterally, and pubic crest anteriorly. Inlet is oval or heart shaped with wider lateral diameter (13·5 cm) than anteroposterior diameter (11·0 cm).

Central part of canal divided into cavity and midpelvis. Roughly circular cross section with diameter of 12·5 to 13·5 cm narrowing down to 10·5 cm between ischial spines.

Outlet bounded anteriorly by pubic arch, laterally by ischial tuberosities and sacrotuberous ligaments and posteriorly by coccyx. Outlet is oval with anteroposterior diameter of 12·5 cm and lateral diameter of 11 cm.

Hence fetus has to enter a tube which is wider laterally at its entrance, becomes round and narrows as it turns through 90° and ends at an opening which is now narrowest laterally. To accomplish this best, movements take place in succession:

1. Flexion. Chin tucked on chest presenting vertex to canal. 95 per cent of births. Engagement of head in canal may have occurred 2 to 3 weeks before onset of labour. Usually occiput lies laterally on left (40 per cent) or right (35 per cent).

2. Internal rotation. As fetus descends head rotates to face sacrum.

3. Crowning. Occiput emerges under symphysis pubis.

4. Extension of head. Perineum sweeps over face as head emerges.

5. Restitution of head. Twisting of neck which occurred at internal rotation now untwists to bring head back in line with shoulders.

6. External rotation of head. This accompanies movement of shoulders as they negotiate birth canal.

7. Internal rotation of shoulders. Shoulders enter inlet obliquely. Anteriorly shoulder passes inlet first then rotates to come under pubic arch.

8. Lateral flexion of body. For posterior shoulder to sweep round curve of sacrum body bends laterally using pubic arch as pivot.

Similar steps occur with other presentations.

Management of normal labour

In Australia 99 per cent of births occur in hospital. Where inadequate facilities exist, Flying Squads are helpful for obstetric emergencies in the home. In Britain 30 per cent of births occur in hospital.

Hospital routine

Admit patient when in labour. Shower. Shave. Collect urine specimen and test. Give enema or suppositories if necessary. Establish that patient is definitely in labour. Monitor interval between contractions and duration of contractions.

General examination carried out. Blood pressure. Abdominal examination to establish lie, presentation, position.

Vaginal examination performed using strict aseptic precautions—cap, mask, hands scrubbed, sterile gown and gloves donned. Vulva swabbed, sterile drapes applied, sterile lubricant used liberally.

First two fingers of right hand inserted gently into vagina with labia separated by finger and thumb of left hand. Care taken to prevent contamination of examining fingers while inserting. Complete examination conducted before withdrawal of fingers.

Examine (1) Vaginal walls; (2) Cervix for amount of effacement; (3) Size of os; (4) Whether membranes still intact; (5) Nature of presenting part; (6) Level of presenting part; (7) Position by determining which fontanelle is palpable.

Management during first stage

Primary power must be allowed to achieve effacement and dilatation. Mother discouraged from bearing down. May be ambulant until contractions are frequent and painful. Uterus exerts less pressure on aorta and inferior vena cava if she lies on her side during later stages. First stage may last several hours and is opportunity for attendants to become familiar with patient and to allay her fears and anxieties.

Record kept of frequency and duration of contractions, 2 hourly temperature, pulse and respirations, 4 hourly emptying of bladder and testing of urine for protein and ketones.

Fetal heart listened for between contractions at half hourly intervals. Rates below 120 or above 160 are suspicious and indicate need for re-assessment of management.

Analgesia, pethidine 100 mg given when os is at 3 cm dilation.

Fluids and light easily digested high calorie foods allowed during 1st stage but only small quantities at a time in case an anaesthetic may be needed later.

Difficulties met with during first stage

1. Fear. Patients should not be left alone. Particularly true for primigravidae. Calm demeanor, sympathetic tone and constant encouragement does much to lessen anxiety.

2. Backache. Standing up and leaning forward over back of a chair helps in early 1st stage. Later, deep massage of sacral regional is effective. Husband can be very usefully employed for this if he is present.

3. Retention of urine. Catheterisation avoided if possible but should be employed without hesitation if bladder becomes distended. Usual careful asepsis essential.

4. Fatigue. Rest encouraged between contractions and sleep encouraged by quiet atmosphere, darkened room, dry, comfortable, well made bed, clean skin, freshly combed hair, warm drink. Pethidine and phenothiazines are good combination.

5. Cramps. Leg cramps can be distressing. May be overcome by straightening limb and dorsiflexing foot and applying firm massage to muscles in spasm.

Management during second stage

Recognition of second stage
Cervix no longer palpable, anus gaping, presenting part appears between gaping labia, perineal bulging.

Other indications of probable transition to second stage, vaginal bleeding—slight bright bleed—rupture of membranes.

Transfer patient to delivery room as soon as second stage is recognised.

Analgesia

Pethidine 100 mg IM. Tranquilisers, e.g. Sparine or Largactil enhance the effect of analgesics and reduce the amounts required. Gas (nitrous oxide) and oxygen useful in middle part of second stage. Oxygen should not be reduced below 30 per cent of mixture. Trilene (Trichlorethylene) 0·5 per cent in air equally good but is cumulative and, used to excess, depresses uterine contractions and neonatal respiratory effort.

Anaesthesia may be required. (See page 107).

Observations

Record:

1. Pulse every ten minutes.
2. Blood pressure every 15 minutes.
3. Frequency and duration of contractions and nature of contraction.
4. Whether uterus relaxes completely between contractions.
5. Whether descent is progressive.
6. Any urine passed tested for ketones.

Fetal observations:

1. Fetal heart beat located between contractions. Record position and rate.
2. Station noted by abdominal, rectal or vaginal palpation.

Evidence of fetal distress. (Page 103.)

Position for delivery

1. Left lateral with right leg supported, either by an assistant or by sling. *Advantages*: ease of access for episiotomy. Greater control of fetal head. More room for manipulation.
2. Dorsal. *Advantages*: no need for change of position between second and third stages. Bearing down is more effective. Mother is usually happier if she can see what is going on.

Episiotomy

If episiotomy to be performed, best done when head down enough to extend and thin perineum. (See page 88).

Attendants and equipment

All equipment for draping patient, clamping and cutting cord, suction, caps, gowns and gloves, swabs, lotions, scissors, catheters and bowls in adequate supplies in readiness. Cot and warmed wraps standing by in care of separate attendant. Articles for resuscitation of baby responsibility of some person other than the accoucheur. Patient draped. Vulva swabbed. Accoucheur scrubbed, gowned, gloved, capped and masked.

Delivery in left lateral position

Accoucheur places left arm round patient's raised right thigh to keep fetal head well flexed until crowning occurs.

Right hand remains passive until crowning and then gently extends head and wipes perineum down over face and under chin.

Each eye wiped from nose with lateral movement with single swab.

Left arm removed from round patient's thigh and head flexed to ensure cord not round neck. About 50 per cent of cords looped at least once round neck. Such loops usually lift easily over head. If not, cut between two clamps.

Observe direction of restitution which will be towards anterior shoulder. Further rotation of head in same direction may be necessary to bring anterior shoulder under symphysis. If shoulder already there rotation not necessary.

Deliver anterior shoulder by cupping head between palms with ulnar borders at level of neck, and applying traction outwards and backwards. Deliver posterior shoulder by changing grip so that thumb and fingers of right hand span baby's occipital region and applying traction forward towards mother's pubis. Gentleness needed at this stage to prevent perineal laceration.

Delivery of trunk and legs usually easily effected by gentle traction with left hand ready to grasp feet and hold baby upside down. Right hand extends head to ensure drainage from nose and mouth.

While mother is turned onto her back babe is held at about the level of her abdomen so that excessive transfer of blood from placenta to infant (babe held low), or from infant to placenta (babe held too high) does not occur.

Mouth sucked out first and then nostrils. Introduction of suction cathether into nasopharynx usually stimulates first inspiration and breathing starts. When mother on her back babe laid on sterile towel between her thighs. Cord palpated. When pulsations cease plastic clamp applied 1 cm from babe's abdomen, and artery forceps applied on maternal side. Cord cut 3 cm from plastic clamp. Babe now handed over to assistant. Sex determined and mother informed.

Management during third stage

Ergometrine usually given IV 0·25 to 0·5 mg as soon as anterior shoulder delivered. This causes contraction of uterus very rapidly. Separation of placenta usually occurs at once and delivery within 10 minutes of completion of 2nd stage.

Classical signs of separation and expulsion rarely seen when erogometrine used. These are lengthening of cord occurring as uterus contracts to globular shape with fundus above umbilicus. Abdomen bulges above umbilicus. Cord does not retract when uterus is moved upwards. Gush of blood at vulva as separation occurs.

Dublin method of delivery commonly employed. When separation and descent has occurred pressure applied to fundus with ulnar border of left hand in downward and backward direction. Placenta taken by right hand and twisted to peel off membranes without tearing them.

More common Brandt-Andrews manoeuvre controlled cord traction consists of applying a Kocher's artery forceps to cord near vulva and applying tension, but not traction, with right hand while left hand pushes uterus upwards by pressing on abdomen suprapubically. Tension applied in line of vaginal axis.

Care after third stage

Care of mother
Examine abdomen. Check if bladder is empty. Ensure uterus is contracted. Examine vagina and perineum. Ensure bleeding absent and repair tears or episiotomy. Estimate total blood loss and record it. Record pulse rate and blood pressure every half hour. Swab vulva and apply large perineal pad. Sponge her and put into clean linen. Encourage rest and sleep. Sedate if necessary.

If after one hour pulse less than 90, blood pressure above 110 systolic and no other contra-indications mother taken to postnatal ward.

Care of baby

As soon as mother has seen and held baby, immediately after birth if possible, baby wrapped in warmed blanket and placed in warmed cot. Immediately note character of respirations, general appearance, colour of skin, any obvious deformities. Report at once cyanosis, pallor, jaundice, lack of movement of any limb, twitches and convulsions, physical defects. Complete detailed examination performed in first hour (see page 121).

Examination of placenta

Estimate amount and colour of chorion. Hold up to light and seek vessels. Note whether such vessels are complete. Suspect succenturiate lobe if vessels end at hole in membranes. Absence of areas of chorion noted and staff of puerperal ward alerted for possibility of haemorrhage.

Placenta inspected measured and weighed. Should be firm and uniformly coloured a deep bluish-red. Undue softness, pallor, white patches, and presence of adherent haematoma noted. Any absent cotyledons reported at once. *Note*: cord length, number and nature of vessels—should be one thin walled vein and two thick walled arteries; Method of insertion into placenta—central, eccentric, battledore, velamentous, presence of true knots.

7. Abnormalities of Labour

Premature rupture of membranes

Normally membranes best intact until second stage. Rupture often occurs in first stage.

When occurring before onset of labour, labour usually starts within 24 hours.

Causes
Poorly fitting presenting part—breech, transverse lie. Hydramnios. Incompetent os. Interference.

Signs and symptoms
Loss of fluid per vaginam. May be sudden, short gush initially. Usually intermittent leaking of small amount. Patient often mistakes it for urine.

Has characteristic odour of liquor.

Micro-examination reveals fetal squames.

Dangers
Premature labour. Before 36 W fetus immature and has reduced chance of surviving. Infection affecting mother and infant.

If fluid loss severe uterus moulds closely round fetus and expulsion is slow and difficult. Uterus may spasm causing reduced placental blood flow and fetal hypoxia. Cord may prolapse.

Treatment
Before 36 W attempts made to prevent onset of labour—rest in bed, sedation with morphia, IV alcohol drip. Antibiotics withheld because of emergence of resistant *E coli* following prolonged administration.

After 36 W encourage onset of labour. If not started within 24 hours set up Syntocinon drip.

Spontaneous preterm labour (premature labour)

Definition
Onset of labour before 37 weeks gestation and after 28 weeks.

Diagnosis
Establish that mother is definitely experiencing contractions, that they are regular and frequent, and that cervical effacement and dilatation are occuring.

Determine cause
50% have a determinable cause. E.g. pre-eclampsia, acute infections, uterine malformation, cervical incompetence, accidental haemorrhage, ruptured membranes, multiple pregnancy, congenital abnormalities.

Contributory factors
Hypertension, maternal malnutrition, anaemia, smoking, previous history of preterm delivery, diabetes.

Prevention
Where contributory factors exist precautions can be taken— correction of anaemia, treatment of hypertension, cervical suture etc.

Treatment
Assessment of fetal maturity and well being and an accurate record of dates essential. Aim is to prolong gestation to a time where fetus has best chance of healthy survival.

It may be that prolongation will add unwarranted risks to mother or infant in which case no attempt made to hinder progress of labour.

Management
1. Inhibition of labour.
2. Stimulation of fetal lung maturity with Betamethasone. Transport mother to hospital with premature infant care facilities.

Inhibition. B sympathomimetic drugs. Ritodrine (Yutopan), Salbutamol (Ventolin), fenoterol (Berotec), terbutaline (Bricanyl).

I.V. normal saline set up, drug added to flask, run in at carefully controlled rate, preferably with automatic monitor and pump.

Ritodine 50–300 μg/min.

Salbutamol 10–50 μg/min. continued up to 48 hours.

Maternal side effects may require reduction of rate— nausea, vomiting, headache, tachycardia, tremor.

Older, less effective methods of inhibiting labour still in use e.g. alcohol infusion, magnesium sulphate injection.

Malpresentation

Definition. Most common presentation is vertex with occiput anterior (OA) and face to sacrum which enables mechanisms to occur with greatest ease. Any other presentation called malpresentation.

Varieties

Occipito-posterior	13 per cent
Breech	3·0 per cent
Face	0·3 per cent
Brow	0·2 per cent
Shoulder	0·3 per cent
Compound Head and hand	
Breech and hand	
Cord	0·5 per cent

Occipito-posterior presentation

Causes. Fifty per cent anthropoid pelvis—antero-posterior diameter of inlet greater than transverse diameter.

Fifty per cent deflexion of head presents greater diameter to inlet which is accommodated more readily in OP position. Occurs more commonly in pendulous abdomen of multiparae.

Diagnosis. Inspection:Abdomen flattened below umbilicus with fundus of uterus prominent above—'pear shaped' abdomen.

Palpation: Back difficult to define. Limbs easily felt all over front of abdomen. Head rarely engaged, occiput and brow at same level.

Auscultation: Fetal heart beat located with difficulty and in early 1st stage usually laterally at level of umbilicus. Vaginal examination when os dilated reveals posterior fontanelle in posterior quadrant of pelvis.

Mechanisms. Head enters inlet OP. Two-thirds rotate head through 135° (long rotation so that face turns towards sacrum and occiput emerges under pubic arch.

One-sixth rotate through 45° (short rotation) so that face turns directly to pubis and emerges face to pubes.

One-sixth rotate so that head lies transversely across pelvis and needs manual or forceps rotation to assist delivery.

Effects of OP presentation. Prolonged labour. Need for forceps in 20 per cent of cases and of CS in 5 per cent with consequent increased risks to mother and infant.

Management. Anticipate long labour. Give adequate sedation. Test all urine specimens for ketones. Anticipate delay in second stage due to prominent ischial spines, inturned coccyx. Examine frequently to determine progress. Do not interfere during first stage. Diagnose arrest early and have anaesthetic and forceps ready for correction.

Maintain fluid and glucose intake, if necessary by IV drip. Keep stomach empty in case anaesthetic needed. Reassure mother constantly.

Delivery. If internal rotation fails and especially if transverse arrest occurs, manual rotation performed followed by application of forceps. Gloved hand inserted and head grasped. Pressure applied externally at inlet level to prevent disengagement and to encourage rotation of anterior shoulder. Ideally rotation brings occiput to pubis. Forceps may be applied when head is transverse or when OA.

Anaesthetic and episiotomy mandatory.

Breech presentation

Definition. Longitudinal lie with buttocks and genitalia presenting. Second most common malpresentation 2·5 per cent of labours.

Varieties

Complete	— Fetus fully flexed.
Frank	— Legs extended up alongside fetal trunk (50 to 70 per cent).
Footling	— One or both hips extended. Foot presenting.
Knee	— Hip extended, knee flexed. Knee presenting.

Causes. Deflexion attitudes especially extended legs which prevent spontaneous version.

More common in multiple pregnancy, hydramnios, prematurity and in fetal abnormality especially anencephaly.

Diagnosis. Palpation:Head palpated in fundus while pelvic area contains soft irregular mass.

Auscultation: Fetal heart beat located with difficulty above level of umbilicus. X-ray or ultrasonography diagnoses completely.

In second stage vaginal examination may reveal details of presenting part, but mistakes often made, anus mistaken for mouth, knee for elbow, foot for hand, coccyx for nose.

Mechanism. Engagement, descent, internal rotation, delivery and external rotation occurs to each part—buttocks, shoulders and head.

Breech engages early, usually before labour. Most common position is left sacroanterior (LSA). Buttocks undergo internal rotation so that anterior buttock passes under symphysis pubis. Lateral flexion of trunk allows posterior buttock to sweep perineum to be delivered.

Shoulders enter canal obliquely. Internal rotation brings anterior shoulder under pubic arch and lateral flexion of neck allows posterior shoulder to sweep perineum in similar fashion.

Restitution of shoulders assists internal rotation of head so that occiput comes under pubic arch. Extension of head assisted by taking body up over mother's abdomen.

Dangers of breech presentation

Anoxia. When head engages cord becomes compressed, fundus is empty and contracts thus compressing uterine vessels and placenta may separate. Time must be allowed for mechanisms and moulding to occur.

Intracranial haemorrhage. Rapid descent of head and insufficient time for rotation and moulding predisposes to cranial compression.

Trauma. Rough or hurried handling by anxious, inexperienced accoucheur may fracture humerus, clavicle, cervical vertebrae, or rupture liver, adrenal glands or lungs. Damage to brachial plexus when twisting body commonly causes Erbs' palsy. Damage to mother mainly laceration of vagina unless adequate episiotomy performed.

Management of breech presentation

External version after 32 weeks often attempted. Should be gentle to prevent complications—ruptured membranes, antepartum haemorrhage, premature labour. Sedation given but not anaesthetic.

Assess size of fetus, presence of fetal abnormalities, presence

of twins, adequacy of pelvis by X-ray pelvimetry in primigravidae.

Decide whether to induce labour early e.g. for large fetus, or
to perform CS, e.g. for elderly primigravida, maternal stature
less than 150 cm, pelvic contraction, or allow to procede to
normal delivery. Breech presentation alone is insufficient to
choose CS as method of delivery.

First stage allowed to procede as for normal labour.

Second stage continues until anus appears between labia minora. Assistance needed from this stage onwards. Episiotomy
performed. Buttock assisted by gentle traction with a finger in
each groin fold. If legs extended they are released by lateral
pressure behind knees.

Fetus now delivered to level of umbilicus and lies with back
uppermost. Anaesthesia may now be induced.

Loop of cord drawn down so that tension on umbilicus is prevented.

Delivery should be complete by another five minutes.

Delivery of anterior shoulder assisted by downward and
backward traction. If difficulty met with, Lovsets manoeuvre
effective. Fetal pelvis grasped and rotated 180° with back
uppermost. This brings posterior shoulder, which is already
within pelvic cavity, into anterior position under pubic arch.
Former anterior shoulder simultaneously enters pelvic cavity.
Rotation back again through 180° brings this shoulder back again
but now under pubic arch.

Delivery of head is crucial stage of delivery. Head kept in full
flexion by allowing body to hang down unsupported (Liverpool
or Burns-Marshall method). Slight suprapubic pressure encourages descent. When hair at nape of neck becomes visible feet are
grasped and traction applied while swinging body up in a wide
arc using pubic arch as a fulcrum to extend neck and deliver
face. Mouth and nose sucked out. Delivery of rest of head can
then be gentle and leisurely to minimize possible cranial damage. Forceps may be used.

Alternative methods of delivering head less commonly employed. Mauriceau-Smellie-Veit manoeuvre consists of straddl-
ing fetal trunk along right forearm, insinuating a finger within
perineum into fetal mouth. Simultaneously left hand placed on
fetal shoulders with middle finger under symphysis against

occiput and other fingers hooked over shoulders. Traction with right hand and pressure with left maintains flexion of head and sweeps face over perineum. An assistant applies suprapubic pressure.

Wigand-Martin method similar but accoucheur applies suprapubic pressure with left hand while right hand applies traction with finger in mouth.

Complications arising during delivery of breech

1. Delay in descent of breech. Reasonable time to allow descent to perineum is 90 minutes. If not, reassess situation. May be necessary to perform 'breech extraction' i.e. bring down a leg manually and apply traction. Hand inserted and leg located, preferably anterior leg, traced to toes and then delivered. Assistant applies fundal pressure. Lovsets manoeuvre performed for delivery of shoulders and Burns-Marshall technique for head.

Patient should be anaesthetized, cervix fully dilated, deep episiotomy cut, bladder and rectum empty.

2. Extension of arms. If delivery refuses to procede past umbilicus arms may be extended. Lovsets manoeuvre performed repeatedly will bring anterior shoulder below symphysis eventually and arm can then be hooked down readily. A further turn through 180° will bring posterior shoulder anteriorly below symphysis allowing delivery of other arm.

Pulling down arms before delivery of shoulders not recommended. High risk of fracture of humerus.

3. Arrest of head. Head may arrest at pelvic inlet, in cavity or at oulet. If at inlet, cause sought—incomplete dilatation of cervix, hydrocephalus, pelvic contraction or deflexed head. Incomplete dilatation treated by incision or stretching under deep anaesthesia. Hydrocephalus or pelvic contraction should be diagnosed before onset of labour and CS performed. If discovered during delivery fetus usually dies and craniotomy performed. Deflexed head may be treated by Mauriceau-Smellie-Veit manoeuvre.

If head rotates to occipito-posterior position delivery attempted by either rotating head to bring occiput anterior and then using Burns-Marshall method or by taking body downwards and backwards and delivering head chin first under symphysis, or by swinging body upwards over mother's abdomen delivering occiput over perineum followed by vault, forehead and face last.

4. Prolapsed cord. Most common with footling presentation. If occuring before full dilatation, CS performed at once. If fully dilated breech extraction may be quicker.

Face presentation

Definition. Head deflexed so that face engages.

Causes. Three-quarters of cases occur by chance, one-sixth because of congenital anomaly, e.g. anencephaly, short neck muscles, goitre or other anterior tumour, remainder because of maternal factors, e.g. pendulous abdomen, flat pelvis. If head enters OP it is likely to deflex as labour continues and uterus compacts fetus more.

Diagnosis. Rarely diagnosed until onset of 2nd stage. On inspection abdomen may be notably pear shaped. On palpation curve of fetal spine interrupted by deep indentation between occiput and back. Occiput very prominent. Vaginal examination reveals irregularities when cervix dilates sufficently, but oedema may obscure ready identification of mouth, nose, orbital ridges.

Mechanisms. These depend on position. When chin (mentum) is anterior, flexion of neck can occur as head negotiates curve of Carus to be delivered face to pubes, but when in MP position internal rotation must occur first to allow this flexion. If mentum remains posterior the fully flexed neck cannot flex any further and arrest occurs.

Effect of face presentation. Diameter presenting are marginally smaller than those in more usual presentation. Submentobregmatic 9·5 cm rather than sub-occipito-bregmatic 10·5 cm. From this point of view face presentation more favourable. However, engagement delayed because more head lies behind submento-bregmatic diameter when it is presenting than when suboccipito-bregmatic presents.

Moulding of facial bones occurs less readily than of cranium and caput likely to be considerable.

Complications. Unlikely unless internal rotation fails to bring chin anteriorly. If chin remains transverse or posterior arrest occurs except with very small babies or anencephalic monsters. Hence, manual rotation essential for successful outcome.

Management. Rotation—manually or with Kiellands forceps for MP positions or with Neville-Barnes forceps for MT positions—needed in 20 per cent of cases. This should be done in theatre where facilities for CS are ready in case of failure.

Brow presentation

Definition. Head neither fully flexed nor fully extended so that brow is foremost. This presents widest diameter of fetal skull for engagement. Supra-occipitomental 13·5 cm.

Cause. Usually engagement occurs before either flexion or extension can happen.

Diagnosis. Palpation may show occiput and chin at same level. Vaginal examination may reveal anterior fontanelle and supra-orbital ridges. Failure to engage is very common.

Management. X-ray to discover cause. In primigravidae CS. In multigravidae may be possible to convert to face or vertex presentation, but should be attempted in theatre where CS can be performed if conversion fails.

Shoulder presentation

Definition. The lie is transverse or oblique.

Varieties. Back anterior—60 per sent; Posterior—40 per cent.

Causes. Large lax uterus of grande multiparae, hydramnios, multiple pregnancy, prematurity, uterine abnormalities—bicornuate uterus, subseptate uterus, large fibroid—placenta praevia.

Diagnosis

Inspection. Wide abdomen,fundus lower than expected.

Palpation fails to locate a pole in fundus and head found in flank.

Auscultation locates heart below umbilicus or fails to locate it at all.

Confirmation by X-ray or ultrasonography.

Mechanism. With a very small premature fetus birth may occur vaginally, but with a full grown fetus normal birth is impossible.

Effects. If untreated fetus dies. Ruptured uterus occurs readily.

Management. Suspicion usually aroused early by inspection of abdomen. External version attempted after 32 W. Often lie is unstable. Version may persist long enough for engagement to occur if done early in 1st stage. If still unstable or if cord prolpases, CS performed.

Where transverse lie occurs with second twin external or podalic version and breech extraction performed.

Cephalo-pelvic disproportion

Definition. Head too big for birth canal.

Causes
Large head as in hydrocephaly or relatively large because fetus is big as in diabetes. Small pelvis because of generally small stature e.g. less than 150 cm, or because of injury, e.g. fractured pelvis, or diseases, e.g. tuberculosis, rickets, congenital dislocation of hip, scoliosis.

Diagnosis
Uncertain until relevant diameters of pelvis and fetal skull can be measured. Former can be measured accurately at any time whereas latter cannot until near to term. Other considerations are degree of laxity of symphysis pubis, amount of moulding skull can take, presentation.

Previous difficulty such as long labour, need for forceps, spastic infant, stillborn infant alert one to possibility.

In primigravidae engagement usually occurs by 37 W. If not, reasons should be sought one of which is cephalo-pelvic disproportion.

Trying to push head into pelvic inlet and measuring degree of overlap is rough guide to degree of disproportion. Munro Kerr's modification of Muller's method is to estimate with two fingers in vagina relative sizes of head and pelvis at same time assessing with thumb degree of overlap above symphysis when the head is pushed down and back with other hand.

Generally speaking a previous normal vaginal delivery indicates probability that cephalo-pelvic disproportion not present.

Treatment
Trial of labour. May await spontaneous onset of labour and follow it through with constant monitoring of progress, descent, dilatation, maternal pulse, blood pressure and stamina, fetal heart rate and mobility, strength, duration and frequency of contractions.

May induce labour with artificial rupture of membranes, followed by cautious use of syntocinon drip and careful monitoring as above.

May decide on CS at outset or resort to CS at any time if maternal or fetal distress occurs or if labour not progressing.

Abnormal uterine action

Normally myometrial contractions in labour are intermittent, regular and coordinated. Each contraction starts at region of tubes and spreads downwards to cervix. Greatest contraction occurs at fundus, least at lower uterine segment. Pain experienced only during height of contraction. Three abnormal states occur, hyperactivity, hypoactivity and incoordination.

Hyperactivity
Myometrium may possess normal regularity and rhythm, but be too forceful causing precipitate labour. Moulding of fetal skull may be forceful and violent causing intracranial haemorrhage.

If obstruction occurs continued powerful contractions causes development of retraction ring and rupture of uterus may follow. Treatment is to deliver fetus at once by forceps or CS.

Tonic contraction or uterine tetany is rare event in which spasm of uterus occurs without relaxation. May be caused by injudicious use of ergometrine e.g. before delivery of unsuspected twin, or if obstructed labour is not treated. The fetus dies due to arrest of placental circulation. Diagnosis by abdominal palpation of firm hard uterus, absence of fetal heart sounds, continuous low abdominal pain.

Hypoactivity
This may be primary or secondary.

In primary hypoactivity (inertia) contractions are regular and intermittent, but of poor quality. Intra-uterine pressure never reaches adequate levels, taking up and dilatation are slow. Patient is not distressed except by length of time it is taking.

Treatment: IV syntocinon makes contractions increase in quality.

Secondary hypoactivity (inertia) arises in second stage in primigravidae especially if descent is held up either with head on perineum or obstructed higher in canal.

Treatment: Forceps delivery or CS.

Incoordination

Initiation of contractions occurs at any point in myometrium or at several points simultaneously. Contractions may be forceful, but fail to achieve taking up and dilatation. Pain severe, colicky, loses its intermittent character. Labour long. Maternal exhaustion may occur.

Often incoordination is accompanied by hyperactivity. Has been termed 'labour in vain'.

Fetal distress

Definition. Term applied to physiological condition of fetus resulting from hypoxia.

Causes

Many conditions reduce amount of oxygen reaching fetus.

Maternal: Anaemia, abruptio placentae, pre-eclampsia, eclampsia, hypertension, cardiac failure.

Fetal: Cord knots, cord round neck, prolapsed cord.

Effects

Hypoxia prevents efficient use of glucose allows accumulation of lactic acid and development of acidosis. Tachycardia occurs initially and later bradycardia. Hyperactivity of intestinal muscle causes premature expulsion of meconium. Hyperactivity of skeletal muscle causes excessive fetal movements.

Diagnosis

Few easy or exact methods of monitoring fetus. Heart beat not easy to locate during contractions and difficult to count accurately. Tococardiography simple and easy to apply, but difficult to interpret. However, fetal heart rate most commonly used means of assessing distress. Rates above 160/minute or below 120/minute persisting between contractions taken to indicate distress.

Other methods: Amnioscopy. Colour and quantity of amniotic fluid determined. Meconium staining taken to indicate fetal distress if liquor was previously clear.

Amniocentesis. Specimen of amniotic fluid aspirated and examined for meconium.

Scalp capillary blood pH. Capillary tube filled with fetal blood and Astrup apparatus used to determine pH. Acidosis if pH less than 7·35. Dangerous degree of acidosis at 7·2 indicating need for surgical interference—CS or forceps.

Prevention
All of antenatal care important in prevention and detection of maternal conditions in which predispose to fetal distress.

Certain conditions in which fetal distress more likely to occur: premature labour, small fetus, disproportion, primigravidae, prolonged labour, excessive use of sedation, maternal hypotension due to dorsal position and pressure on inferior vena cava, epidural or caudal anaesthesia. Avoided by lateral position.

Treatment
Rapid separation of fetus by application of forceps or by CS. Administer oxygen to mother.

Obstetric emergencies

1. Prolapsed cord

Definition. Cord lies distal to presenting part after membranes rupture.

Causes. Malpresentation, especially complete breech, transverse lie, footling and knee. Hydramnios. Multiple pregnancy. Less common in primigravidae because engagement occurs earlier than in multigravidae.

Danger. Engagement compresses cord and cuts off placental circulation. Fetus dies if untreated.

Diagnosis. Cord felt or seen in vagina.

Treatment. Immediate CS, but until patient reaches theatre, replace cord in vagina; place mother in Sims position; elevate buttocks on pillows; elevate foot of trolley; keep presenting part from engaging with gloved hand in vagina until patient anaesthetised and ready for CS.

2. Ruptured uterus

Definition. Uterus tears usually at a line of fibrous tissue from previous scar.

Causes. Almost always multiparae in labour with either obstructed labour, previous CS scar present especially classical vertical scar, or injudicious use of oxytocic agents.

Occasionally occurs during internal version or forceps delivery through incompletely dilated os.

Rupture during pregnancy rare. More likely if pregnancy occurs soon after previous scar incurred, e.g. CS, perforation during D and C, placental abnormality during previous pregnancy—percreta, increta, acreta—recent myomectomy.

Signs and symptoms. During pregnancy. Pain and tenderness over uterus. Increasing shock. Shoulder tip pain.

During course of normal labour. Constant abdominal pain. Worse during contractions. Failure to progress. Gradual onset of shock with rising pulse rate and falling blood pressure. Occasionally bleeding is severe and collapse is very rapid.

During obstructed labour. Constant severe abdominal pain. Retraction ring palpable. When lower uterine segment tears pain changes to dull ache and contractions cease. Shock develops rapidly.

Treatment. Restore circulating volume. Perform CS. Usually hysterectomy performed. Occasionally tear repaired.

3. *Amniotic fluid embolus*:

Definition. Entry of amniotic fluid into veins of uterus causes pulmonary embolus, pulmonary oedema, hypofibrinogenaemia, haemorrhage.

Cause. Hyperactive uterus with prolonged forceful and frequent contractions. Associated with excessive use of oxytocic agents. May accompany ruptured uterus.

Signs and symptoms. Dyspnoea. Cyanosis. Tachycardia. Bubbly respirations. Crepitations in all lung fields. Hypotension. Bleeding without clot formation.

Treatment. Oxygen. Fibrinogen IV. Transfusion of fresh blood. Deliver infant by forceps if birth has not yet occurred. Corticosteroids IV e.g. Solucortef 500 mg statim and bd for 5 days. Broad spectrum antibiotics IV.

4. *Obstetric shock*

Definition. Sudden collapse during or shortly after third stage.

Causes. Usually post partum haemorrhage.

Others—rupture of uterus, amniotic fluid embolus, clots in uterus, inversion of uterus.

Signs and symptoms. Pallor. Tachycardia. Hypotension. Cold clammy skin. Rapid shallow respirations at first, later deep and sighing. Restlessness.

Treatment. Rest. Calm. Elevate foot of bed. Replace circulating volume preferably with cross-matched blood, but emergency group O Rhesus negative, plasma, haemacell, 5 per cent dextrose or rheomacrodex until blood is ready. Oxygen.

Abnormalities of third stage

Primary post-partum haemorrhage: (PPH)

Definition. Loss of more than 300 ml blood (or any amount causing deterioration in patient's condition during first 24 hours after delivery.)

Causes. Uterine—clot remaining from ante partum haemorrhage, presence of fibroid, rupture, inefficient contraction of myometrium.

Placental—retention of part or all of placenta, cotyledon, succenturiate lobe, placenta accreta, increta, percreta.

Laceration of cervix, vagina, perineum, clitoris.

Blood coagulation disorder.

Diagnosis. Bleeding. Failure of uterus to contract and stay contracted. Soft, boggy uterus. Shock.

Prevention. Expect and prepare for PPH in grande multiparae, previous history of PPH, presence of APH where fibroids present.

Give ergometrine 0·5 mg IV when anterior shoulder born.

Treatment. Encourage uterus to contract. Remove retained products (see below). If 3rd stage completed, remove clots, instal syntocinon drip IV 20 units per litre running at 30/minute delivers 40 micro units per minute.

If bleeding from cervix or vagina, search for bleeding site and ligate.

Retained products:
If anything remains within uterus after delivery myometrium unable to contract fully and arterioles not closed off, hence haemorrhage occurs.

Causes. Retained placenta, cotyledon, membranes, clots.

Treatment. Empty uterus.

If placenta partially separated, uterus rubbed up to obtain contraction and gentle traction applied to cord while pushing uterus upwards to prevent inversion.

If no separation obvious, separation may be effected by obtaining firm contraction and then compressing fundus between thumb and fingers. Fingers have to dig down deeply to obtain grip (Crede's method). Is painful and should be tried once only.

Manual removal performed if simpler methods fail. General anaesthetic given. All aseptic precautions taken. Gloved hand insinuated into vagina with palm uppermost. Fingers locate edge of placenta and strip it up while other hand on outside of abdomen presses uterus against stripping fingers, and prevents distension and tearing of lower uterine segment.

Complications of manual removal
Ruptured uterus. Infection. Haemorrhage if placenta is accreta.

Clots easily removed manually and uterus caused to contract by rubbing up and administration of ergometrine to prevent relaxation.

Inverted uterus:
Extremely rare complication due to cord traction while uterus atonic or to Crede's method of expulsion.

Signs and symptoms. Severe pain in lower abdomen, rising pulse rate, falling blood pressure, haemorrhage may be severe. Uterus not palpable abdominally. Placenta usually still adherent, protrudes through cervix.

Treatment. Replace uterus with pressure of gloved hand against inverted fundus. Treat shock.

8. Obstetric Operations

Version

Definition. Changing the lie of fetus so that more favourable part presents.

Terms. *Cephalic version*: Head is brought to lie over inlet;
Podalic version: Breech is brought to lie over inlet.

Method

External: Purely external forces are applied to mother's abdomen.

Internal: Purely internal forces are applied.

Bipolar: Partly external and partly internal forces are used.

Reasons. To convert a breech or transverse lie to one of cephalic presentation.

Time. Not before 34th week because lie is unstable and will revert.

External version

Method. Patient must be relaxed. Sedation usual, e.g. pethidine 100 mg. Abdomen and operators hands dusted with talcum. Patient lies comfortably on back with foot of bed elevated on 15 cm blocks. Breech eased upwards out of pelvis. Pressure applied to head and breech to encourage fetus to somersault forward into head down position.

Difficulties. Breech may not disengage. If legs extended, somersault may be impossible. Abdominal muscles may be too rigid.

Contra-indications. Pre-eclampsia. Hypertension. Previous CS. Twins. Known uterine abnormality.

Dangers. Abruptio placentae. Ruptured membranes. Premature labour. Looping of cord round limb.

Precautions. Avoidance of anaesthesia. Relaxation of mother. Avoidance of undue force.

Internal podalic version

Indications. Transverse lie especially of second twin.

Object. To convert to breech prior to breech extraction.

Method. With cervix fully dilated, mother deeply anaesthetized and with full aseptic precautions, hand introduced and limb located. Heel identified and leg pulled down slowly and gently. External hand applies upward pressure on head.

Dangers. Rupture of uterus. Damage to fetus. Introduction of infection.

Bipolar version. Rarely performed and CS in safer.

Induction of labour

Definition. Artificial stimulation to cause onset of labour.

Indications. Maturity of pregnancy; Pre-eclampsia; Eclampsia; Hypertension; Accidental haemorrhage; Fetal abnormality; Intra-uterine death; Fetal distress; Falling oestriol levels; Meconium staining of liquor; Maternal diseases—cardiac, renal, diabetic. Rhesus incompatibility.

Methods. (1) Medical; (2) Surgical.

Medical

(i) Oxytocin (ii) Prostaglandin E_2.

(i) Oxytocin given IV, sublingually, or intranasally will cause uterine contractions. Latter two methods less reliable and less amenable to control and rarely used. Most common means is IV.

Complications. Anaphylactic reaction in sensitive persons. Tonic contraction of uterus. Accidental haemorrhage. Rupture of uterus.

Administration. IV drip installed. Very dilute oxytocin solution used initially. 2 units (Syntocinon) in 1 litre 5 per cent dextrose delivered at 15 drops per minute gives 2 micro units of oxytocin per minute. Rate increased every ten minutes until 45 drops per minute reached or until contractions occur every 3 to 5 minutes and last 60 to 90 seconds.

If no contractions at 45 drops per minute concentration of Syntocinon solution increased to 8 units in 1 litre 5 per cent dextrose and rate reduced to 15 drops per minute, i.e. 8 micro units per minute.

Drip rate increased by increments of 5 drops per minute every

10 minutes until labour starts or until contractions are regular and of satisfactory force. Drip rate then maintained at constant rate or reduced if necessary or stopped altogether.

Drip stopped after 10 hours to prevent fluid overload.

(ii) Prostaglandin E_2. Prostaglandins ripen cervix and increase sensitivity to oxytocin. Probably vaginal slow release pessary will be available soon. Presently oral (sublingual) tablets in use. 0·5 mg hourly × 10 will induce labour within 36 hours in 50 per cent of cases. If followed by oxytocin. I.V. and amniotomy success is about 95 per cent.

Surgical

Artificial rupture of membranes (ARM) (amniotomy). Rupture of forewaters most commonly. Often used with Syntocinon drip. Some obstetricians prefer to anaesthetize patient and perform procedure in theatre. More often performed under sedation only.

Method. Patient placed in lithotomy position. Antiseptic preparation carried out. Two fingers of gloved and well lubricated hand inserted and membranes within cervix stripped gently: Kocher or Goodwins forceps guided by tip of finger to grasp membranes and tear a hole. Hole may then be enlarged with finger.

Rupture of hindwaters less common. With same precautions, Drew-Smythe cannula inserted through external os and passed behind fetal head stripping membranes in its path. When tip is at level of fetal neck stilette is pressed home and ruptures membranes.

In both methods 200 to 500 ml fluid drain off.

Monitoring. Fetal heart rate monitored every five minutes for first hour after ARM. Mother's pulse and blood pressure taken half hourly. Liquor observed for blood and meconium staining. Amount, colour and odour of liquor noted.

Complications

Failed induction. Occurs in 20 per cent when Syntocinon drip not added to procedure and 5 per cent when both methods combined.

Success related to careful selection of moment to try. Best when gestation advanced, cervix is ripe, engagement is secure.

Prolapse of cord. More likely with forewater rupture because head must be displaced to allow escape of liquor. Also in breech presentation.

Haemorrhage. Traumatic or abruptio. Trauma may be to mother or fetus. Fetal bleeding diagnosed by laboratory test. May indicate need for CS. Abruptio may result from sudden release of liquor especially in hydramnios.

Sepsis. Very likely to occur if induction fails. Hence antibiotics started if labour has not started by 24 hours. Combined therapy used e.g. penicillin and streptomycin, to prevent emergence of resistant strains.

Pulmonary Embolism. Very rare. Usually fatal. (See page 90).

Once ARM performed obstetrician is committed to deliver child within 72 hours. 80 per cent deliver vaginally within 24 hours. Only 5 per cent fail to deliver within 48 hours. These usually come to CS.

Episiotomy

Definition. Incision into perineum to enlarge introitus at time of delivery.

Indications
To forestall tearing of perineum which may extend to anal sphincter. To prevent vaginal or clitoral damage especially in malpresentation or when forceps to be applied. To prevent delay in delivery due to stiff unyielding perineum.

Site
Incision starts at midpoint of posterior fourchette and may extend in the midline (median) or mediolaterally to within 2 cm of anus.

Time. Incision not made until head distends pelvic floor. This time may be anticipated and local anaesthetic infiltrated 5 minutes before.

Technique
Two fingers inserted to protect head. Sharp, long scissors inserted between fingers. Cut made quickly, cleanly and in one go. Repeated little nibbling cuts make a ragged wound, difficult to repair and more likely to bleed.

Repair

Patient placed in lithotomy position, swabbed and draped. Operator scrubbed, capped, gowned and gloved. Vagina anaesthetized with 1 per cent lignocaine and inspected for lacerations and bleeding. Apex of episiotomy located and suture tied to secure vessels entering from apex. Muscle and deep layers opposed and secured with No. 00 interrupted catgut. Mucous membrane and skin edges accurately matched and secured with either a subcuticular continuous suture or interrupted sutures of 00 catgut.

Area inspected to ensure bleeding controlled. Finger inserted into rectum to ensure that sutures have not been placed through rectal mucosa.

Forceps

Use

To grasp fetal head so that traction or rotation can be applied without injury.

Indications

Whenever it is considered that delivery should be speeded up, e.g.:

1. When second stage extends beyond one hour in primigravidae or half an hour in multigravidae. Common causes are transverse arrest in midcavity, maternal exhaustion, unyielding perineum, persistent OP position.

2. When it is desirable to deliver quickly because of poor maternal condition such as coexisting disease, cardiac, renal, hypertension, pre-eclampsia, ante partum haemorrhage.

3. When fetal distress is detected.

4. To deliver aftercoming head in breech presentation.

5. Transverse arrest needing rotation of head to OA.

Conditions necessary for forceps application

1. Cervix fully dilated
2. Fetal head fully engaged
3. Bladder and bowels empty
4. Membranes ruptured
5. Patient adequately anaesthetized

Common types of forceps and their uses

1. Neville-Barnes forceps. Invented by Barnes. Modified by Neville so that axis traction more easily applied. Blades have cephalic curve to fit fetal head and pelvic curve to fit curve of Carus. Ideal for traction when fetal head is OA and sagittal suture is directly anteroposterior. Unsuitable for rotating head because of pelvic curve. Axis traction attachment originally invented to aid traction when forceps applied to head high in birth canal. Such application no longer used, but attachment useful when head is in mid canal.

2. Kielland forceps. Cephalic curve of blades as in Neville-Barnes type, but pelvic curve is minimal. Shank (between blades and handle) long and straight. Sliding type lock. Handles with shoulders for applying traction without compression.

Lack of pelvic curve makes these highly suitable for rotating head from OP or OT positions.

3. Wrigley's forceps. Short shank. Light construction. Suitable for application when head low in canal, e.g. for final lift over perineum when mother tired or uterine contractions getting poor.

Method

Mother placed in lithotomy position. Area swabbed. Catheter passed. Drapes positioned. Pudendal block anaesthesia generally employed. Pelvic examination performed to ensure vertex presentation, favourable position and station, cervix fully dilated, membranes ruptured. Manual rotation of head attempted to bring OA. Forceps applied one blade at a time until locking device and handle come together without force being applied.

Episiotomy cut if difficulty experienced in application of forceps or if rotation to be performed.

Forceps may be used to deliver in OP position especially if mother has a contracted pelvis. In face presentation with mentum anterior forceps may be applied direct.

Traction is applied intermittently matching contractions. Excessive force dangerous.

Complications of forceps delivery

1. Injuries to baby. Properly applied blades protect fetal skull. Improperly positioned may caused bruising, depressed fracture, facial nerve palsy.

2. *Tearing of cervix, vagina or perineum*. Adequate episiotomy at correct time obviates tearing of vagina or perineum. Cervix least likely to be damaged when fully dilated.

3. *Haemorrhage*. If tearing occurs.

4. *Failed forceps*, i.e. attempt to deliver with forceps has been unsuccessful.

Causes:

1. Cervix not fully dilated. Give morphine 15 mg and promazine 50 mg and wait for labour to progress to vaginal delivery or try again when cervix fully dilated.

2. Misdiagnosis of presentation. Head is OP or face presenting. Check and correct position.

3. Mid-pelvic contraction or outlet contraction. CS may be required.

Vacuum extraction (Ventouse)

Apparatus consists of bottle from which air sucked out by pump, controlled by pressure gauge and a suction cup connected to bottle by tubing. Traction applied to suction cup by chain inside the tubing. Cups of various sizes available.

Method of use
Lithotomy position. Pudendal block anaesthesia. Appropriate size of cup applied to presenting scalp avoiding fontanelles. Air pumped from bottle to total pressure of 800 g/cm^2. Suction increased gradually over 5 to 10 minutes before traction applied. Traction used synchronously with contractions.

Advantages
Compression of skull avoided. Laceration of vagina less likely. Can be used during first stage once cervix is more than 5 cm dilated. (Said to aid full dilatation when delay has occurred.)

Disadvantages
Caput succedaneum marked and may take a week to subside. Cephalhaematoma more common. Laceration around edge of cup if applied for longer than 30 minutes.

Amnioscopy

Definition. Inspection of amniotic fluid through intact membranes via special endoscope.

Requirements
Cervix dilated to at least one finger to admit endoscope.

Purpose
To detect abnormal colour of amniotic fluid as in post-maturity, erythroblastosis, fetal abnormality.

Technique
Patient placed in lithotomy position, swabbed, draped. Endoscope with obturator in situ inserted through external os. Obturator removed and light adjusted to illuminate amniotic fluid.

Dangers
Accidental rupture of membranes. Premature labour. Damage to cervix. Introduction of infection.

Amniocentesis

Definition. Aspiration of sample of amniotic fluid.

Purpose
To assess amount of bilirubin present and hence degree of haemolysis of fetal blood in iso-immunisation (see page 64), sphyngomyelin/lecithin ratio to assess fetal maturity (see page 125 and 136) to determine level of alpha fetoprotein which rises steeply in neural tube defects-anencephaly, spina nifida, collection of foetal cells for culture and determination of enzyme manufacture.

Method
Lumbar puncture needle inserted through mother's abdomen above umbilicus on side opposite to fetal back. Up to 5 ml fluid aspirated. Amount of bilirubin directly porportional to light absorption at 450 m microns.

Dangers
Haemorrhage. Passage of fetal red cells into maternal circulation with consequent worsening of immune reaction.

Scalp capillary blood

Definition. Sampling of fetal blood during labour.

Purpose
To determine placental gas exchange indirectly by estimating pH of fetal blood and thus to measure fetal distress.

Technique
After membranes ruptured, endoscope passed through os with end resting against fetal scalp. Capillaries dilated with ethyl chloride spray. Silicone cream applied to prevent spreading of blood. Incision made with guarded blade limiting depth of cut. Blood collected into heparinised plastic capillary tube and subjected to pH analysis at once by Astrup pH meter.

Interpretation
pH of fetal capillary blood usually between 7·25 and 7·35. Below 7·2 indicates dangerous degree of acidity and need for rapid delivery.

Laparoscopy and culdoscopy

Definition. Method in which pelvic organs can be viewed without a major incision. Laparoscopy performed via an endoscope introduced through abdominal wall; culdoscopy via posterior fornix into pouch of Douglas. Illumination best provided by Cold Light System. Light source separate from endoscope. Light conveyed through flexible fibreglass cable.

Purposes
(1) To view pelvic organs for differential diagnosis of ectopic pregnancy, ruptured luteal cyst, adherent ovaries, ovarian cysts; (2) Cautery of fallopian tubes.

Technique
Performed under general anaesthetic. Patient placed in Trendelenburg position for laparoscopy and in lithotomy position for culdoscopy, to allow abdominal organs to slide away from pelvis. Abdominal cavity distended with carbon dioxide or helium. Endoscope introduced via small incision.

Disadvantages
Equipment very expensive. Much experience needed to interpret what is seen through the endoscope. Some discomfort experienced from pneumoperitoneum. Possibility that adhesions

induced by pneumoperitoneum. Pre-existing pelvic adhesions may make viewing impossible.

Symphysiotomy

Definition. Division of symphysis pubis to allow vaginal delivery especially in pelvic outlet contraction. Very rarely used nowadays except in France and in some developing countries when medical aid is difficult to get. Occasionally for obstructed labour with head engaged and cervix fully dilated.

Method
Performed under general anaesthetic. Transverse supra-pubic incision to expose symphysis. Cartilage cut down to subpubic ligament.

Dangers
Great strain thrown on vestibular structures. Tearing may involve urethra and bladder.

Advantages
Additional 4 cm of transverse diameter gained in pelvic outlet allowing application of forceps and easier vaginal delivery.

Caesarean Section(CS)

Definition. Delivery via incisions through anterior abdominal wall and uterus.

Types:
(1) Classical; (2) Lower uterine segment (LUS).

Classical: Longitudinal incision through muscle of upper uterine segment.

LUS: Transverse incision through thin fibrous tissue of LUS.

Classical CS safer in inexperienced hands when emergency operation necessary. Operation of choice when CS performed for impacted transverse lie, when fibroids distort anatomy or when speed is essential in very ill patient. LUS CS best for elective operation. Scar heals firmly and rarely ruptures in subsequent pregnancies. Greater risk of severe haemorrhage, however, especially if incision carried too far laterally into uterine vessels or if tearing extends incision. Other complications less likely—

peritonitis, ileus, adhesions, placental adhesion—acreta, increta, percreta—in subsequent pregnancies.

Indications for CS
1. Previous CS.
2. Placenta praevia and abruptio placentae.
3. Cephalopelvic disproportion.
4. Malpresentation.
5. Obstructive tumours—ovarian, myomata, pelvic osteomata.
6. Pre-eclampsia.
7. Maternal disease.
8. Fetal distress.
9. Prolapsed cord.
10. Abnormal uterine action.
11. Failure to labour after surgical induction.
12. Failed forceps.
13. Older primigravida.

Most common reasons are first three—about two-thirds of all CS. Percentage of deliveries varies in different countries. Australia about 4 per cent; England 8 or 9 per cent; USA 5 per cent.

Occasionally CS followed by hysterectomy, e.g. for ruptured uterus, multiple myomata, placenta acreta.

Technique of Classical CS
Blood cross matched. Drip installed. General anaesthetic given. Vertical paramedian incision one third above umbilicus two-thirds below. Abdominal organs encouraged to fall away with Trendelenburg position and packed off. Uterine incision made midline. Placenta incised in 40 per cent of cases—ignored. Lower limb grasped and baby gently extracted and cord divided between clamps. Baby handed immediately to paediatrician.

Ergometrine 0·5 mg given IV. Placenta and membranes removed completely. Wound closed in 3 layers.

Technique of LUS CS
Blood cross matched. Drip installed. General anaesthetic given usually. Occasionally performed under spinal. Subumbilical midline incision or suprapubic transverse incision. Latter preferred for cosmetic reasons. Scar hidden in pubic hair. Loose peritoneum covering LUS divided and pushed down. Bladder

identified and occasionally surgeon places identifying coloured sutures to mark bladder and prevent accidental injury.

Transverse incision made as low down as possible through LUS. Membranes bulging through incision ruptured. Fluid aspirated. Head manoeuvred so that face presents at incision. Delivery effected, occasionally with Wrigley's forceps and fundal pressure by assistant. Ergometrine 0·5 mg IV given as head delivered. Placenta and membranes delivered.

LUS sutured in two layers. Internal layer excludes decidual layer. Bleeding from venous sinuses at angles of incision may be troublesome. Peritoneum closed without tension.

Complications

1. Paralytic ileus: Very common, especially after classical CS. Nil orally until bowel sounds return. Distension eased by regular aspiration via naso-gastric tube.

2. Haemorrhage: From placental site or from angles of LUS incision. Hence need for cross matched blood before starting.

3. Wound dehiscence: Abdominal distension strains incision. More likely with classical incision.

4. Chest complications: Pulmonary embolus, atelectasis, pneumonia.

5. Late complications: Ventral hernia, abdominal adhesions and obstruction.

Destructive operations

Definition. Operations on fetus, dead or grossly abnormal, to enable vaginal delivery. (Rarely performed. CS preferred).

Types

Craniotomy. Opening into skull and draining ventricles to reduce bulk in hydrocephaly.

Decapitation. Impacted shoulder presentation. Head severed at neck so that trunk and head may be delivered separately.

Cleidotomy. Division of clavicles to reduce width of shoulders.

Evisceration. Enlarged abdomen of some monsters may prevent delivery. Incision into abdomen and removal of contents may allow delivery.

Tubal ligation

Definition. Method of contraception which prevents access of spermatozoa to ova and passage of ova to uterus.

Indications
Where further conceptions would endanger the health of mother or where no further family will be required.

Number performed limited by willingness of surgeons to spend time operating and devoting hospital bed to non-essential case.

Disadvantage of operation is irreversibility.

Method
Under GA tubes clamped and ligated with nonabsorbable suture. Various techniques used to ensure nonpatentcy of lumen, e.g. excision of 2 to 4 cm and burying stumps, cauterizing stumps, plicating tubes and double ligation.

Time of operation
At time of CS or two days after delivery or two months after delivery.

Obstetric anaesthetics and analgesics

Requirements of safe analgesics
Relieve pain without clouding consciousness or depressing uterine action. Must not depress fetal respiratory centre. Must be non-toxic to mother and fetus.

Commonly used sedatives and analgesics

Phenothiazine derivatives. Chlorpromazine (Largactil), 50 mg IM, promethazine (Phenergan) 25 mg with pethidine 50 mg IM and promazine (Sparine) 50 mg IM. Produce drowsiness, relieve nausea and vomiting and potentiate analgesics. Do not depress fetal reflexes.

Diazepam (Valium, Ducene) 10 to 20 mg IM, Oxazepam (Serepax, Serenid D) 20 to 50 mg orally reduce anxiety and produce amnesia. Crosses placenta readily, but without noticeable effects post-natally.

Pethidine (Meperidine, demerol) 100 to 150 mg IM.

Excellent analgesic. Patient often sleeps during labour. Increases rate of cervical dilatation, hence shortens first stage. Depresses fetal respiratory centre, hence not given in late first stage or during second stage.

Morphine 10 to 15 mg IM. Excellent analgesic, but depresses fetal respiratory centre severely. This effect most marked in premature infants. Used only in early first stage.

(Respiratory depression in newborn can be reversed to some extent with Nalorphine (Lethidrone) or Levallorphan (Lorfan). Both antagonise morphia and pethedine induced respiratory depression, but themselves are sedative and analgesic, 0·25 mg into umbilical vein or 0·5 mg IM.)

Barbiturates used rarely nowadays. Have no analgesic effect and unpredictable sedative effects. Frequently produce depression of all fetal reflexes.

Inhalational agents

Nitrous oxide. Good analgesic. Does not depress maternal or fetal respiration. Does not reduce uterine contractions. Safe for self-administration. Mixtures with air not recommended because oxygen content of mixture less than the required 20 per cent and will produce fetal hypoxia. N₂O/oxygen mixtures can be guaranteed to contain at least 30 per cent oxygen.

Entonox apparatus approved by Central Midwives Board uses N₂O/O₂ 50·50 mixture. Piped N₂O and O₂ can pass through regulatory valve preventing reduction of O₂ below 30 per cent or above 50 per cent.

N₂O/O₂ mixture recommended in late 1st stage and in 2nd stage regularity of contractions allow anticipation of next contraction and inhalation can start 4 or 5 breaths before pain starts.

Trichlorethylene (Trilene). Good analgesic and good sedation. Tends to cause anaesthesia when administration prolonged. Given by various types of machine for self-administration by mother, e.g. Tecota Inhaler, Cyprane Inhaler, Emotril Inhaler which deliver concentration of vapour in air ranging from 0·22 per cent to 0·54 per cent. Lower concentrations quite effective if pethedine also given.

Passes placenta readily, but does not seem to harm fetus in any way.

Methoxyflurane (Penthrane). Inhaled in 0·35 per cent concentration in air produces excellent analgesia, better than trichlorethylene or 50 per cent N_2O. Cardiff inhaler delivers 0·35 per cent and cannot produce anaesthesia when used intermittently.

Anaesthetic agents

Local anaesthesia

Extremely rich nerve supply to uterus, vagina and pudenda. Motor sympathetics to uterus derived from level of T6 to L2. Sensory from uterus enter spinal cord at levels T11 and 12. Parasympathetic fibres to cervix, which allow cervical dilatation, come from S2, 3, 4. Somatic sensory nerves to vagina, clitoris, labia and perineum derived from sacral plexus via inferior rectal, perineal, dorsal nerve of clitoris, plus ilioinguinal and genitofemoral nerves from lumbar plexus.

Various levels of interruption of sensory impulses

1. Regional infiltration of peritoneum. Lignocaine 1 per cent up to 20 ml during late 2nd stage prior to episiotomy. Anaesthesia sharply localized, persists for 45 to 60 minutes. Immediate post-partum repair of episiotomy needs no further infiltration.

2. Pudendal block (plus regional infiltration). Long needle and director placed by guiding fingers in vagina to lie medial and inferior to tip of ischial spine. 10 ml 1 per cent lignocaine injected each side and further 5 ml each side into perineal tissues. Useful for episiotomy, forceps application, final stages of normal delivery, repair.

3. Paracervical block. Injection of 5 ml into each lateral fornix of 0·25 per cent bupivacaine. Stops pain of cervical dilatation. Danger of absorption into uterine vessels feeding placenta and causing fetal depression.

4. Caudal and epidural anaesthesia. Introduction of anaesthetic into space outside dura mater via either caudal hiatus between 5th sacral vertebra and coccyx or directly between L1-2 or L2-3. Caudal hiatus safer and easier in unskilled hands. Special needles through which fine catheter can be passed allow for small repeated doses of anaesthetic to maintain analgesia for days if necessary.

Bupivacaine 0·5 per cent or 0·25 per cent 5 to 10 ml (repeated 3 hourly if necessary) most commonly used. Mepivacaine 1·5 per cent and Lignocaine 2 per cent also used. Bacterial filter should be attached to tube if it is to remain in situ for long.

Used for prolonged labour, maternal cardiac or respiratory disease, trial of labour, pre-eclampsia, forceps. Some hospitals advocate its use for all deliveries unless definitely contra-indicated. Contra-indications—haemorrhagic disease or anti-coagulant therapy, local sepsis, shock, hypotension, hypo-volaemia.

Close monitoring essential following epidural as all painful stimuli abolished and warning of complications must be sought from other parameters, e.g. (a) Hypotension: Patient should lie on side to prevent obstruction of venous return. Hypotension treated with IV fluid load, e.g. litre N. saline in 30 mins.

(b) Headache—as in spinal anaesthesia. Treated by analagesics and maintenance of horizontal position.

(c) Convulsions. Too large amount of local or inadvertent injection into epidural vein. Preceded by twitching.

(d) Urinary retention. Careful observation and relief by catheter when noted.

Contraindications to epidural

(a) Local sepsis.

(b) Blood disorders.

(c) Hypotension.

(d) Previous CS.

5. Spinal or subarachnoid block. Anaesthetic introduced via lumbar puncture needle into subarachnoid space or theca. Through L3-4 space anaesthesia of perineum and inner thighs but not of legs generally—'saddle block'. Drugs used: Procaine HCl 50 mg dissolved in 2 ml CSF. Needs up to 15 minutes to work. Cinchocaine HCl 0·5 ml of hyperbaric solution with 0·5 ml CSF.

Amethocaine 4 mg in 2 ml 5 per cent dextrose. Useful for mid-forceps application or whenever painless birth is indicated. Does not depress fetus. Relaxes perineal muscles. Accelerates cervical dilatation.

Disadvantages: causes fall in BP and subsequent fetal hypoxia unless precautions taken—avoid dorsal position with 15° tilt to left or full lateral position, keep legs elevated, ensure adequate blood volume, give oxygen. Headaches may be severe and unresponsive to treatment.

Contra-indications: Disproportion; Placenta praevia; Non-engagement. Hypotension. Hypovolaemia.

General anaesthesia

Should be administered only by qualified anaesthetist experienced in obstetric anaesthesia or under his guidance. Deaths occur from inhalation of vomitus and from inadequate correction of hypovolaemia.

Preparation of patient should include—

Keeping stomach empty or emptying it if insufficient time since last intake; induction of anaesthesia with head *elevated;* premedication of atropine 0.6 mg; intravenous line installed beforehand; small quantity thiopentone, 250 mg, used IV to induce; cricoid pressure maintained until endotracheal tube installed.

Thiopentone (Pentothal) depresses fetal respiration hence kept to a minimum. Advantageous if actual delivery delayed for up to 10 minutes after using thiopentone by which time much will have been metabolized.

Pancuronium for muscle relaxation affects fetus least.

Nitrous oxide and oxygen 2:1 believed by many to be best anaesthetic for obstetric work. Non-toxic to mother or fetus; rapidly reversible; good analgesic.

Halothane depresses uterus. May predispose to post partum haemorrhage.

Methoxyflurane. Good analgesic. Supplements N_2O/O_2 anaesthesia. Good muscle relaxant.

Oxytocics

Drugs which cause uterine contraction.

(1) Oxytocin; (2) Syntocinon; (3) Ergometrine.

Oxytocin

Manufactured in hypothalamic cells. Transported to posterior lobe. Stored. Released in increasing amounts during pregnancy. Release stimulated by irritation of cervix (and by suckling postpartum). Action on uterus to produce muscular contractions. Used for induction of labour together with surgical ARM, continuous intravenous infusion (see page 94); to augment contractions in uterine inertia; to bring about rapid contraction of uterus in 3rd stage and thus reduce incidence of PPH; to stop PPH.

Syntocinon

Synthetic octapeptide with similar properties to natural oxytocin.

Used for same reasons. Given IV or IM. Continuous IV infusion of low concentration for induction of labour. High does IV infusion for induction in fetal death.

Contra-indications to oxytocin or Syntocinon: previous CS, malpresentation, cephalo-pelvic disproportion, grande multiparity.

Ergometrine
Alkaloid extract from ergot. Given IM or IV causes prolonged tetanic spasm of uterus. IV injection of 0·5 mg causes spasm in 30 seconds which lasts 30 minutes. IM injection produces spasm in 10 minutes which lasts 3 hours. Prevents PPH, but incidence of retained placenta increases. Most common use is in 3rd stage. Also used for bleeding of abortion. Can be given orally, but control of absorbed dose lessened.

9. The Puerperium

Puerperium

Definition: Puerperium extends from end of 3rd stage for about two months.

Physiology
Involution of uterus, ligaments, pelvic floor, vagina, perineum.

Oestrogen and progesterone levels fall rapidly to non-pregnant levels. Without their support uterine muscle bulk rapidly diminishes to former size. Immediately after 3rd stage fundus extends to umbilicus. Thereafter it recedes into pelvis at rate of 1 cm a day. Barely perceptable by 14th day.

Lochia. Vaginal discharge following birth. Lochia rubra first 3 to 4 days; red watery discharge. Lochia serosa next 5 to 8 days; pale yellowish colour. Lochia alba for 9 to 14 days; colourless watery discharge. Gradual lessening colour and amount.

Subinvolution:
Term applied when uterus fails to return to former size. Lochia heavier and grades into PPH.

Causes: Retained products. Endometritis. Fibroids. Missed twin. Chorion carcinoma.

Signs and symptoms. Pyrexia. Bulky tender uterus. Offensive lochia. Swab shows anaerobic gram negative organisms and anaerobic streptococci.

Treatment: Mild cases—oral ergotrate (ergometrine malleate) 0·5 mg t.d.s. Others—penicillin 1 million units/day and sulphadimidine 2 g statim and 1 g q.q.h.

D and C may be performed, but great care necessary. Uterine wall soft and friable. Easily perforated. Blunt curettage gently performed.

Other changes noted in puerperium

Pulse. Tends to be slow, less than 70.
Temperature. Slight elevation for 24 hours.
Constipation. Common for up to 1 week.

Urine. Diuresis with output exceeding intake for 4 to 5 days.
Breasts. Colostrum excreted for 1st 3 days until oestrogen levels fall (see later).

Immediate check after 3rd stage

Cervix, vagina, clitoris, labia, perineum examined for bleeding and for tears. Episiotomy sutured. Major tears repaired and examination of rectum and anus made. Especial care taken to ensure anal sphincter intact. No. 00 catgut used to effect repairs. Second and third degree tears repaired in layers. All sutures placed without tension. Damage more likely to be sustained if baby large, OP position, application of forceps, precipitate labour, in primigravidae, when tear occurred in previous deliveries.

Other puerperal complications

Haematoma of vulva
May be massive. Can be cause of hypovolaemic shock. May need evacuation, vaginal pack, transfusion, antibiotics.

Colporrhexis
Rupture of vaginal vault. Usually at lateral or posterior fornix. Often result of inexpert application of posterior blade of Kielland's forceps.
Treatment. If rupture through into peritoneal space, laparotomy necessary to repair and control haemorrhage. Hysterectomy may be needed.

Vesicovaginal fistula
Rare. May be due to long continued pressure by fetal head. More likely due to instrumentation. Bladder catheterized and drained for 10 days. Fistula repaired in two layers.

Recto-vaginal fistula
Rare, provided tears adequately examined and repaired fastidiously. May occur if suture of episiotomy penetrates rectal wall and operator fails to check.

Ruptured uterus
Almost always preceded by previous classical CS. Occasionally

due to obstructed labour especially in grande multiparous. Rarely from too vigourous application of syntocinon without adequate monitoring.

Signs and symptoms. Rapid development of shock with pain, pallor, rapid feeble pulse, restless anxiety, falling blood pressure, cessation of contractions and fetal heart beat.

Occasionally 'silent' rupture occurs with no shock or pain. If tear occurs through lower segment bleeding may be minimal.

Treatment. Laparotomy. Repair of LUS tears. Hysterectomy for others.

Acute inversion of uterus

Very rare if ergometrine used at proper time.

Causes. Inexpert application of cord traction, large lax uterus of grande multiparity.

Degrees. First—fundus felt through cervix. Second—fundus and body lie within vagina. Third—whole organ protrudes from introitus. Often placenta is adherent.

Consequences. May be: severe shock, bleeding and death; strangulation and gangrene of uterus; chronic prolapse; infection.

Treatment. General anaesthetic. Manual replacement. Ergometrine to achieve contraction. If unsuccessful—laparotomy, stretching and incision through constriction ring (Bandl's) and correction via abdomen and perineum simultaneously.

Puerperal infection

Definition. Infection of birth canal or part thereof with subsequent spread via blood stream. Notification compulsory in many countries. Various rules apply. Notification necessary in England if temperature of 38°C, occurs within 14 days. Less common now, but for centuries was most common cause of maternal death.

Organisms

Almost always mixed growth of organisms. May be commensal from genital or gastro-intestinal tracts, or exogenous from attendant's hands, respiratory tract etc., or from instruments, catgut etc. Especially dangerous organisms—haemolytic group A streptococci, gram negative intestinal bacteria, *Clostridium welchii*. Very common organisms—anaerobic streptococci.

Prevention

Strict attention to environmental factors—clean wards, beds, furniture. Sterilized linen. Special air filtration for especially vulnerable areas—delivery rooms, nursery.

Constant awareness of danger by all personnel with high index of suspicion and social conscience regarding skin infections, sore throats, etc.

Strict aseptic procedures well learned and rehearsed as to become second nature.

Signs and symptoms

Depends on grade of infection with history of recent delivery or abortion.

Grade 1. Mild. Infection confined to birth canal. Patient not greatly incommoded. Pyrexic to 39°C. Settles within one week.

Grade 2. Moderate. Infection spreads beyond birth canal to involve parametrium, tubes and ovaries or pelvic veins.

Patient has low abdominal pain, tenderness PR and PV. Pyrexia to 40°C. Pulse rate to 120.

Grade 3. Severe. General peritonitis. Patient gravely ill with general abdominal pain, distension, tenderness, paralytic ileus, continuous pyrexia, tachycardia, dehydration from vomiting.

Grade 4. Very severe. Septicaemia.

Treatment

Differentiate from other causes of infection, e.g. mastitis, urinary and upper respiratory tract infections. Take vaginal swabs and blood for culture.

Immediate start of antibiotics. Combinations of penicillin and sulphonamide effective for almost all infections. Cultures and sensitivities available in 24 hours may demand alteration to drug of choice, Metronidazole 500 mg t.i.d.

Commonly ampicillin 500 mg given 6 hourly plus combined sulphonamides, e.g. Sulphatriad (sulphadiazine, sulphamerazine, sulphathiazole) 2 g initially and 1 g four hourly thereafter. Drugs continue for 7 days or until 2 days after symptoms and signs disappear.

In Grade 3 and 4 infections. Fluid and electrolyte balance need correction. Antibiotics given IV at start. Methicillin may replace penicillin to give better cover against staphylococci.

Complications
Pelvic abscess. Salpingitis. Deep vein thrombosis. Pulmonary embolus. Metastatic abscesses in kidney, liver, lungs, brain.

Venous thrombosis

Incidence
About 3 per cent in Australia. 1·5 per cent in U.K. 0·1 per cent in developing countries. Superficial vein thrombosis ten times more common than deep vein thrombosis.

Cause
Primary cause unknown. Predisposing factors: varicose veins, immobility, infection, pressure on inferior vena cava by uterus when mother lies supine. Prolonged pressure on calf veins if post-partum sedation allows patient to lie immobile for long periods. Possibly anaemia and dehydration play a part.

Signs and symptoms
Pain in leg increased by pressure or by dorsiflexion of foot (Homan's sign). Slight pyrexia. Superficial vein thrombosis— inflammation and cellulitis along course of affected vein.

Occasionally no local signs or symptoms until intensive search made following pulmonary embolus—chest pain, haemoptysis, shortness of breath, tachycardia, cyanosis. Occasionally massive occlusion of veins and spasm of femoral artery causes puerperal white leg (phlegmasia alba dolens) with severe pain, swelling , coldness, pallor and, rarely, gangrene.

Prophylaxis
Full mobility as soon as possible especially after CS. Anticoagulation before CS—subcutaneous calcium heparin 5000 units continued post-operatively for 3 days. Electrical stimulation or pump massage of calf muscles throughout operation. Support under ankles to prevent pressure on calves.

Treatment
Heparin. Either 10 000 units IV 6 hourly or continuous IV drip set to deliver 5000 units in 100 ml normal saline or Hartman's solution every 4 hours. Blood taken for clotting time every 24 hours and dose adjusted to maintain clotting time at about 20

minutes. After 7 to 10 days, anticoagulation changed to phenin-
dione (Dindevan) 100 mg or dicoumarin (Warfarin) 2 to 15 mg
daily in single dose. Prothrombin time taken daily and maintained at about 30 per cent of normal. (Normal value established
by testing control subjects daily.)

Dangers of anticoagulation therapy watched for constantly—
haemorrhage into joints, gastro-intestinal and urinary tracts,
submucous layers, from nose, into skin. Occasionally post-
partum haemorrhage occurs.

Patient confined to bed with firm bandage applied to leg.
Analgesics given freely.

Psychiatric disturbance

Occurrence
0·1 per cent. More common in primigravidae.

Types
None peculiar to pregnancy or puerperium. Often history of
psychiatric disturbance before or between pregnancies, or family
history. Personality problems accentuated during pregnancy and
especially when demands made by new baby have to be shoul-
dered by mother alone.

Depression common. Suicidal impulses more frequent and
often successful during pregnancy. Schizophrenia less common.
Hypomanic attacks rare, but more likely in first two weeks after
delivery.

Rejection of doctor, nurse, husband, baby may occur. Belief
that baby is abnormal may cause attempts on its life.

Treatment
Sedation with chlorpromazine (Largactil) up to 100 mg daily or
similar preparations for hypomania. Anxiety with agitation—
diazepam (valium) or oxazepam (Serepax). Psychiatrist may
order electroconvulsive therapy for acute depressive illness.

General supportive care away from other patients temporarily.
Visitors strictly limited and controlled. Patient not left alone at
any time.

Post-partum haemorrhage (PPH)

Definition. Primary PPH occurs within 24 hours of delivery

(See page 91). Secondary PPH—any undue bleeding occurring after first 24 hours.

Causes

Most commonly retention of remnants of placenta, membranes. or blood clots. Occasionally infection. Rarely, hypofibrino-genaemia following deep vein thrombosis. Rarely chorion carcinoma.

Treatment

Ergometrine 0·5 mg IM may be sufficient. If not, digital examination of uterus under general anaesthetic necessary. Gentle curettage followed by ergometrine takes care of almost all cases.

Curettings should always be examined by pathologist if bleeding is late and persistent in order to exclude chorion-carcinoma.

Sheehan's syndrome

Definition: Necrosis and atrophy of pituitary gland. Very rare.

Cause

Thrombosis of vessels of anterior lobe (pituitary portal system) following episode of hypotension.

Signs

Failure to lactate. Later, indications of lack of secretions from anterior pituitary lobe develop—hypothyroidism, failure to ovulate or menstruate, degeneration of breast tissue.

Treatment

Hormone replacement therapy.

The breasts

Throughout pregnancy glandular tissue, blood and lymphatic vessels multiply under influence of increased oestrogen and progesterone. Prolactin from anterior pituitary causes secretion of milk. Prolactin suppressed by oestrogen. During first three days post-partum, oestrogen levels fall rapidly while prolactin levels rise.

Oxytocin causes 'letting down' of milk from glands into lactiferous ducts. Oxytocin secreted reflexly following stimulation of nipples either manually or by suckling.

Colostrum secreted until levels of prolactin rise. Contains 6 per cent protein, 2·5 per cent fat, 3 per cent carbohydrate. Rich in gamma globulins. Milk contains 1 per cent protein, 3·5 per cent fat, 7 per cent carbohydrate.

Advantages of breast feeding
Warm. Sterile. Right constituents in ideal state of suspension. Morbidity and mortality lower in breast fed babies. Closer maternal/baby relationship. Psychologically satisfying to mother.

Disadvantages
Social mores make breast feeding an embarrassment for many women. Desire for independence from infant for periods longer than three hours denied. Father cannot share in feed preparation and administration.

Establishment of breast feeding
Baby put to breast three or four times in first 24 hours. Thereafter every 3 to 4 hours until good production and flow established, then 'on demand'.

Mother should not be rushed, ridiculed or nagged. Prolactin production easily inhibited by fear, anger, disgust.

Inhibition of lactation
In developed countries half the mothers do not wish to breast feed. Their wishes should be established before the birth. Easier to suppress lactation from outset than after it has started. Tight binders and fluid restriction condemned. Maintenance of oestrogen level (ethinyloestradiol 0·1 mg t.d.s. for 3 days then daily for 6 days), gradual withdrawal and not putting infant to suckle is generally sufficient. Bromocriptine (Parlodel) 2·5 mg orally b.d. × 14 days, relieves congestion, prevents engorgement and stops milk production.

Breast engorgement
Definition. Presence of oedema and obstruction of veins and lymphatics because milk not removed fast enough.
Causes. Balance between production and removal not yet established. Occasionally ducts blocked with colostrum or sebum.
Signs and symptoms. Painful, tense, swollen breasts, with flattened nipples.

Treatment. Depends on severity.

If mild—gentle washing with warm water, stroking breast towards nipple with gentle pressure from soapy hands, apply babe to suck and expressing milk remaining thereafter.

If severe—analgesics, even pethidine at night, and temporary suppression for 24 to 48 hours with ethinyloestradiol 0·1 mg b.d.

Good supporting brassiere essential.

Breast infection

Definition. Invasion of breast segment by organisms, usually *Staphylococcus aureus*, via cracked or abraded nipple, which may progress to abscess formation and axillary lympha-denopathy.

Signs and symptoms. Pyrexia, tender nipple, tender, reddened area radiating from nipple to periphery.

Later hot, painful lump develops with tender nodes in axilla.

Treatment. In early stage, before lump has developed—antibiotic (methicillin, cloxacillin or similar to combat peni-cillin-resistant strains of staphylococci). Suppress lactation with ethinyloestradiol.

When abscess has developed, radial incision under GA, drain-age tube inserted for 3 days. Suppress lactation. Start antibiotics only when effective drainage is established. Starting antibiotics before then causes cessation of liquification process and persis-tent hard lump with much fibrous tissue develops in which infec-tion may persist for months. (Antibiotoma.)

Differential diagnosis of breast abscess

1. Swollen, painful 'axillary tail' of mammary tissue without infection.

2. Galactocoele. Segment of breast tissue fails to excrete milk.

3. Carcinoma.

Post-natal check

Usually 6 weeks after delivery. Lochia should have stopped. Enquiries made regarding menstruation, discharge, breast feed-ing. Blood pressure measured. Urine tested. Weight taken.

Physical examination made including heart, lungs and abdomen, but major attention centred on vulva, vagina, cervix and uterus.

Note healed lacerations, any prolapse, laxity of levator ani, stress incontinence. Take smears for cytological examination. Note position of uterus. If retroverted and subinvoluted correct with Hodge ring pessary and re-examine in 8 weeks.

Persistent red lochia demands D and C and examination of scrapings to exclude chorioncarcinoma.

Give patient every opportunity to ask questions. Often valuable information regarding sexual matters, contraception, family planning, important at this time.

10. Care of Neonate

Immediate care

Eyes

During delivery eyes wiped with sterile swabs. In many hospitals drops applied to eyes, e.g. silver protein.

Airway

Baby held suspended with head down to facilitate drainage of amniotic fluid from lungs, mouth and nose. Suction applied to mouth, pharynx, stomach, nostrils, briefly in that order. Pass suction tube into stomach to exclude oesophageal atresia.

Avoid excessive or prolonged sucking. If meconium passed prior to delivery, laryngoscope passed to ensure none clinging to larynx or in trachea. Suction to nostrils often stimulates first breath. Suction should be intermittent and short duration.

Cord

Clamp applied to cord close to skin and cord cut 2 cm distal to clamp. Cord stump squeezed to evacuate blood. Inspected for presence of 3 vessels. Covered with dry dressing and binder.

Warmth

Baby wrapped in sterile cotton cover and blanket, shown to mother who may want to hold it for a few minutes, then placed on side with head slightly lowered. Taken to a quiet, warm, draught free area. Undisturbed for the next half hour or so.

Excessive vernix caseosa wiped away most easily soon after birth. Becomes more tenacious if allowed to dry.

Assessment of Apgar score

Points allotted for heart rate, respiratory effort, muscle tone reflex irritability and colour. Points are 0, 1 or 2 for each.

Heart rate: Absent 0; Below 100 1; Over 100 2.

Respiratory effort: Absent 0; Slow 1; Good 2.

Muscle tone: Flaccid 0; Feeble 1; Good 2.

Irritability: Nil 0; Grimace 1; Crying 2.

Colour: Cyanosed or pale 0; Body pink 1; Completely pink 2.

Assessment made at 1 minute and 5 minutes after birth.

Score of 7 or over indicates healthy baby.

Score of 5 to 6 at one minute improving to 7 to 10 at five minutes satisfactory.

Score below 5 at 5 minutes needs immediate and continuing intensive care.

Immediate requirements

Asphyxiation needs emergency correction. Establish airway, ventilate adequately, correct acidosis, maintain circulation.

If baby fails to breathe after all liquor, meconium, lanugo, vernix, mucous blood sucked out, frog breathing tried for one minute, then mask for one minute, then intubation and positive pressure oxygen.

Frog breathing—with nostrils held and oxygen catheter in corner of mouth, mouth is opened then closed with fingers under chin compressing floor of mouth. This increases intraairway pressure and stimulates respiratory reflexes. Mask and positive pressure oxygen does similarly. Mouth to tube respiration also. In all except a few infants five to ten puffs enough to initiate spontaneous respirations.

Correction of acidosis. Umbilical vein cannulated. Sodium bicarbonate 1 mEq/ml diluted with half volume of 10 per cent glucose. Mixture = 0·67 mEq/ml up to 15 ml injected slowly. (5 ml per kg birth weight.) If resuscitation prolonged, 5–15 ml 0·67 m Eq/ml repeated every 5–10 mins.

Adrenaline. Persistent bradycardia, less than 50/min inspite of correction of acidosis and oxygenation, may respond to IV adrenaline 2 ml 1: 10 000 solution.

Hypovolemic shock—pale, immobile child with B.P. less than 30 mmHg needs infusion of 30–50 ml saline, plasma or blood.

It may be possible to aspirate sufficient from vessels of placenta using a heparised syringe and injecting directly into umbilical vessel.

Narcotic antagonists. May be useful if mother received narcotics during last 4 hours of labour.

Morphia, pethidine, omnopon best avoided for this reason. Antagonists naloxone (Narcan) 0·01 mg/kg, average dose

0·03 mg or nalorphine (Lethidrone) 0·25 mg/kg average dose 0·75 mg given IV.

Glucose. Check blood glucose with Dextrostix. If low, below 30 mg per cent, 5 ml N saline with 5 ml 10 per cent dextrose given IV.

Other measures sometimes needed: external cardiac massage, blood transfusion, intracardiac adrenaline, IV glucose 1 to 2 ml 50 per cent solution, narcotic antagonists, nalorphine or levallorphan.

Examination

Warm room, warm hands, good light necessary.

Appearance
Note colour. Should be pink all over. Look especially for pallor, cyanosis, jaundice.

Respirations
Normally irregular at 40 to 50 per minute. Normally noiseless. Note rate, any dyspnoea, prolonged expiratory phase, noises either on inspiration or expiration, rib or abdominal muscle retraction during inspiration.

Heart
Auscultate. Count rate. Normally 120 to 140. Sinus arrhythmia very common. Rate up to 160 if crying.

Measurements

Weight. Average 3500 grammes ± 750 g at full term. (Less 125 g/week born before 40 weeks.)
Length. Average (vertex to heel) 50 cm.
Head circumference. Average 35 cm.
Temperature. Rectal 37°C.
Head. Feel tension of fontanelles. Observe indications of moulding, cephalhaematoma, plagiocephaly. Regard symmetry and placement of ears. Use auroscope to ensure patent meati.
Open eyes. Note symmetry, pupil size, whether equal and responding to light. Look for cataract.
Regard nose for free airway. Note any discharge.
Open mouth to observe for bruising, cleft palate, presence of

teeth. Test for 'rooting reflex' with finger against cheek.

Pass nasogastric tube into stomach to ensure patency of oesophagus.

Arms

Feel pulses—axillary, brachial, radial. Regard palms for single palmar crease (Down's syndrome). Count fingers. Open fist to avoid missing extra digit folded into palm. Place a finger in palm to elicit grasp reflex.

Umbilicus

Check that clamp is firm and that no bleeding has occurred.

Spine

Look for spina bifida, naevus, hair tuft or sinus.

Genitalia

Examine scrotum for presence of testes. Examine prepuce for phimosis. Expose urethral meatus for hypospadias. Prepuce usually adherent at birth. Hydrocele common and subsides over first 6 weeks.

Examine females for presence of vaginal orifice. Note size of clitoris; enlargement may indicate adreno-genital syndrome.

Anus

Ensure anus patent. If in doubt insert small lubricated catheter.

Lower limbs

Exclude congenital dislocation of hips using Ortolani's click test. With hip and knee flexed to 90° hold thigh with thumb against lesser trochanter and middle finger against greater trochanter steady pelvis with other hand and abduct thigh. If joint subluxed it will slip back into acetabulum with pronounced click. Repeat for other hip.

Palpate femoral pulses. Compare amplitude with brachial. Difference may indicate coarctation of aorta. Observe number of toes, absence of talipes. Check equality in length of limbs.

Abdomen

Note normal protruberance of abdomen. Auscultate for bowel sounds. Palpate and percuss for liver and spleen. Palpate for kidney size. Left usually palpable.

Reflexes

Test for Moro reflex by elevating head with child recumbent and allowing head suddenly to fall back. Arms and sometimes legs will abduct and then close into body as if clutching. Primitive fall reflex. Disappears by 12 to 20 weeks.

Glabella tap. Tap forehead where root of nose lies between eyes. Causes blink each time if performed at about 5 second intervals. Rapidly fatigues if repeated at one second intervals.

Blink reflex elicited by sudden clap of hands together—crude hearing test.

Automatic stepping. (Walking reflex) Support child with feet just touching a hard surface.

Rooting reflex and grasp reflex already referred to.

Common peculiarities mistaken for abnormalities

White spots on nose: Sebaceous excretion which clear in few weeks.

Mongolian blue spot: Lumbar or sacral bluish discolouration. Fades gradually. Reassure mother.

Pallor of hands and feet with pinkness everywhere else: Common result of vasomotor instability which soon settles. Also cause of mottling generally.

Vaginal discharge milky or bloody: Results from oestrogen activity. Settles within a few days.

Hydrocele; Fullness of scrotum. Subsides in 6 to 12 weeks.

Respiratory Distress Syndrome (RDS)

Also called hyaline membrane disease. Hypoxia most common cause of neonatal mortality and morbidity. One cause is RSD.

Definition. Syndrome in which alveoli fail to aerate or fail to remain aerated when dilated by positive pressure.

Cause

Immaturity of lung physiology. Failure to secrete a substance, surfactant, which prevents over distension of alveoli on inspiration and complete collapse of alveoli on expiration. Normally increase of surfactant production occurs about 32 week.

Infant's first breath needs pressure of 40 to 60 mm water. Thereafter breathing needs no more than 20 mm pressure.

In RDS every breath needs 40 to 60 mm H_2O or more to inflate alveoli which promptly collapse completely on expiration.

Detection before birth

Amniocentesis performed. Ratio of lecithin to sphyngomyelin determined. Before 34 weeks ratio is 1: 1. At term ratio is 20: 1. Ratio bears close relationship to RDS. If ratio is 2: 1 disease unlikely to occur.

Susceptible infants: Predominantly premature.

Others—maternal diabetes, CS, pre-natal asphyxiation due to maternal hypotension and maternal hypoxia.

Diagnosis

Floppy baby. Respiration: 60+. Sternal and costal retraction, grunting expirations.

Cyanosis may or may not be present. If present even in high O_2 environment, prognosis poor.

On auscultation: poorly heard breath sounds. Increased heart rate.

X-ray shows well expanded thoracic cage with ground-glass appearance of lungs.

Treatment

Nurse undisturbed in Isolette with O_2 at sufficient concentration to prevent cyanosis. Correct acidosis. Maintain clear airway. Assist ventilation, if blood gas estimations show persistent hypoxaemia or hypercarbia.

Lower ambient O_2 to level which maintains adequate pO_2. Prolonged high O_2 causes development of fibrous tissue in submucous layers. If baby can be kept alive long enough, maturation of lung tissue occurs. Administer human plasminogen 1 ml IV at birth.

Prevention

Dexamethasone 4–16 mg in divided doses. IM injection: must be given 48–24 hours before delivery.

Salbutamol (Ventolin) 8 mg 6 hourly orally given to mother during 24 hours before delivery or 500 mg IM within 3 hours of delivery or 250 mg IV during second stage.

These regimes markedly reduce incidence of R.D.S. in premature infants.

Other causes of respiratory difficulties

Obstruction of airway—choanal atresia, laryngeal stenosis, Pierre-Robin syndrome (cleft palate and retraction of lower jaw).

Infection—pneumonia.

Inhalation of blood or meconium (amniotic fluid not dangerous as it is absorbed readily unless heavily contaminated.)

Congenital malformations—diaphragmatic hernia, cardiac malformations.

Treatment: O_2; assisted respiration if necessary; antibiotics if necessary; correction of electrolyte and acid-base upsets; adequate glucose intake. Correction of causative factors.

Birth injuries

Injuries to head

Causes. Too rapid or too severe moulding due to:
   a. Precipitate labour
   b. After-coming head in breech
   c. Malpresentation
   d. Large baby or small pelvis
   e. Inexpert application of forceps
   f. Engorgement of cerebral vessels due to anoxia, making vessels more vulnerable.

Prevention. Recognition of risk factors. Early decision to assist delivery where necessary with episiotomy and forceps or CS. Extreme care during delivery especially in malpresentation.

Types of injury. Minor—moulding; caput succedaneum; cephalhaematoma; facial paralysis.

Major—depressed fracture; intracranial haemorrhage.

Moulding. Head flexible at suture lines and accommodates to fit better the birth canal. Cranial bones may overlap to considerable extent without internal damage provided process takes place slowly enough. Reduction of moulding occurs in first 48 hours.

Caput succedaneum. Localised oedema within a compression ring probably applied by cervix after rupture of membranes. Site of swelling depends on presentation. Disappears in first 48 hours.

Cephalhaematoma. Haemorrhage under pericranium. Pericranium adheres at suture lines, therefore haemorrhage confined to area overlying one flat bone, most commonly parietal. May be multiple.

Recognition. Fluctuant swelling. Confined to area correspond-ing to flat bone. Occasionally linear fracture demonstrated. Does not subside in 48 hours. Peripheral calcification after one week.

Course. Gradual absorption and disappearance. Occasionally calcification causes asymmetry which may take 12 to 18 months to mould.

Occasionally volume of haemorrhage sufficient to cause anaemia and jaundice from haemolysis.

Treatment. Konakion injection 1 mg IM.

Facial paralysis

Cause. Pressure on one or more branches of facial nerve as it emerges onto face anterior to ear and passes over ramus of man-dible. Pressure occurs from forceps or mother's pelvis.

Recognition. Immobility of one side of face during crying. Inability to close completely one eye while asleep.

Course. Spontaneous recovery within a week or so.

Treatment. Protection of cornea until recovery.

Major head injuries:

Depressed fracture

Rare occurrence in cephalo-pelvic disproportion. Spoon shaped or furrow depression in parietal or frontal bones. No treatment required unless localizing signs develop from intracranial haemorrhage. Elevation with ventouse suction apparatus gives good results without need for surgery.

Intracranial haemorrhage

Site of ruptured vessel. (1) Cerebral veins entering superior sagittal sinus, ruptured by excessive moulding, causing subdural haemorrhage. Rare. (2) Great cerebral vein (vein of Galen) where it is joined by right and left basal veins and enters the straight sinus. This area is particularly vulnerable to stresses and strains. Right and left halves of tentorium cerebelli join falx cerebri. These are rigid, taut sheets of fibrous tissue. Excessive moulding tears one or other sheet and disrupts veins with bleed-ing into subdural space which easily breaks through into sub-arachnoid space.

Recognition. Child depressed at birth with pallor, lethargy.

Later, fontanelles may be tense and bulging. Later—convulsions, dilated non-reacting pupils excessive activity, tremulousness, high pitched cry.

Diagnosis. Subdural tap—needle inserted into lateral corner of anterior fontanelle.

Lumbar puncture revealing evenly blood stained CSF.

Prognosis. Whole spectrum of end results seen, from early death, through survival with cerebral palsy to apparent complete recovery.

Treatment. Nurse in intensive care unit with oxygen, head elevated position, gavage feeding sedation and anticonvulsants if necessary, Konakion 1 mg IM.

Injuries to nerves
   1. Facial nerve—see above.
   2. Brachial plexus. Excess traction on head to deliver shoulders of big baby or traction on trunk to deliver head in breech presentation. Damage to upper roots of plexus causes Erb's palsy, to lower roots Klumpke's paralysis.

Erb's palsy—arm extended at elbow, pronated and flexed at wrist—porter's tip position.

Klumpke's paralysis (rare)—wrist drop and paralysis of hand muscles.

Treatment. Correct position. Place limb in neutral position and maintain with splint and bandage.

Prognosis. Usually recovery complete because axons not torn, merely compressed by oedema from damaged sheath.

   3. Sciatic nerve. Occasionally damaged by inexpert IM injection. Consequence is severe—paralysed, wasted lower limb.

Fractures
Clavicle. Humerus. Femur. Not common. Occur where pressure has to be exerted to effect delivery; e.g. femur in extended breech, humerus in extended hand beside aftercoming head, clavicles when performing Lovset's manoeuvre.

Treatment. Clavicle and humerus. Immobilize arm by enfolding it against chest with sling. Femur—gallows traction.

Neonatal infections

Potent cause of neonatal deaths. Neonates capable of manufacturing additional polymorphs in response to infections, but mechanism for disposing of phagocytosed organisms appears to remain incompetent.

Susceptible infants

Premature. Following prolonged labour, difficult forceps or premature rupture of membranes. Diabetic mother. Dysmature infant. Those who need instrumentation—intubation, umbilical vein cannulation. Those needing exchange transfusion. Those with congenital abnormalities involving incomplete skin closure—spina bifida, ectopia vesicae, pilonidal cyst. Those with signs of fetal distress.

Signs and symptoms

May be minimal, non-specific and vague, e.g. failing to thrive, with vomiting, diarrhoea, lethargy.

Pyrexia uncommon. Hypothermia more common.

Irritability, twitching, convulsions, Hepatomegaly. Splenomegaly. Jaundice. Petechiae.

Investigations

Full blood examination especially white cell count and erythrocyte sedimentation rate. Urinalysis.

Serological evaluation for syphilis, toxoplasmosis, rubella and cytomegalic inclusion disease.

Microscopic examination and culture of swabs from nose, rectum, umbilicus, throat. Lumbar puncture for protein, glucose, chloride.

X-ray chest and abdomen.

Biochemical studies—blood sugar, urea, potassium, sodium, calcium, bilirubin.

Blood group. Rh. factor. Reticulocyte count. Coomb's test.

Treatment

(1) Antibiotics pending definitive results from culture and sensitivity tests, e.g. combination of penicillin and Kanamycin, or methicillin and Kanamycin. Should always be given IV or IM; (2) Isolate in temperature controlled environment with piped oxygen and humidification. 'Isolette' serves admirably; (3) Instal IV line for fluids and glucose.

Specific infections

Congenital syphilis

Rare where routine exclusion of maternal disease performed before 16 to 18 weeks and antisyphilis treatment instituted in positive cases. Common in some developing countries.

Signs. Large, boggy placenta. Hepatosplenomegaly, small infant, skin lesions especially on palms and soles, osteochondritis, periostitis.

Diagnosis. IgM fluorescent treponemal antibody test (IgM FTA). VDRL test on cord blood. X-ray long bones.

Treatment. Crystalline penicillin 125 000 units b.d. for 10 days IM.

Gonococcal conjunctivities

Most hospitals have some routine installation eye drops—silver nitrate, penicillin, erythromycin, tetracycline, sulphonamides, hence, conjunctivitis uncommon.

Signs. Severe conjunctivitis, blepharitis, thick yellow or copious watery discharge.

Diagnosis. Immediate Gram stain of fresh swab and culture on chocolate agar under increased CO_2 concentration.

Treatment. Crystalline penicillin 125 000 units b.d. for 10 days IM. Usual to cleanse eyes and instil erythromycin ointment.

Specialist ophthalmic examination advised for all cornea after conjunctivitis.

Non-specific conjunctivitis

Often due to silver nitrate if arising within 24 hours of instillation—not pussy and without blepharitis and oedema. Settles spontaneously.

Other causative organisms. Staphylococcus aureus, proteus, streptococcus, pneumococcus, pseudomonas.

Treatment. Cleanse. Instil Neosporin drops after taking swabs for micro, culture and sensitivities.

Bullous impetigo

(Pemphigus neonatorum).

Cause. *Staphylococcus aureus.* Rare since introduction of hexachlorophene (pHisoHex: Hibitane).

Signs. Erythematous areas rapidly progressing to blisters which break down to raw weeping areas, similar to burns in appearance.

Treatment. Isolate and quarantine contacts for 5 days. Bathe with pHisoHex. Methicillin 50 mg q.i.d. IM or Nafcillin 20 mg b.d. IM

Escherichia coli infections

Infant intestines rapidly colonized with E. *coli*. Spread of organisms to eyes, throat, umbilical cord stump occurs readily especially in sick infants. Often organism resists more usual antibiotics. Most strains sensitive to ampicillin, neomycin or polymixin (Colymycin).

Thrush

Cause. Colonization of mucous surfaces and moist skin areas with monilia (*Candida albicans*—a yeast.)

Source of organisms. Present in vagina of 25 per cent women. Readily spread from contaminated hands to bottles, teats.

Signs. Greyish-white raised patches on mucous surfaces leave raw bleeding surface if rubbed off. Most commonly distributed over cheeks, gums, tongue, fauces. Occasionally over napkin area, anus, vagina, penis. May cause substantial diarrhoea.

Prognosis. Harmless in otherwise healthy baby, but indicates need for greater vigilance with hygiene. Can be extensive throughout intestinal and respiratory tracts of premature children and those already ill for other reasons, in whom it may contribute towards death.

Treatment. Oral Nystatin 100 000 U 6 hourly for 10 days. Nystatin cream to napkin area if required. Look to hygienic precautions with hands, napkin disposal, feeding bottles, teats, nipples.

Virus infections

Rubella

Congenital deformities result when contracted during first trimester—cataract at 5th to 7th week, deafness at 8th to 9th week, cardiac anomalies 5th to 10th week.

Diagnosis of infection in mother. Rising titre of rubella antibodies in two samples of blood taken two weeks apart. Abortion offered.

Neonate may continue to excrete virus in all secretions for many months. Should be isolated while in hospital to prevent spread of infection to staff. No specific treatment.

Herpes simplex

Can be fatal in neonates. Virus spreads from mother or attendant with a 'cold sore'. Viraemia causes febrile illness, hepatomegaly, vomiting, diarrhoea. In severe cases, thrombocytopenia and petechiae may be seen.

Jaundice

Cause

Breakdown of red cells releases unconjugated bilirubin which is bound to albumin in plasma, carried to liver, conjugated there and released in bile. If this sequence fails, skin becomes visibly yellow when bilirubin reaches level of 5 mg per 100 ml blood.

Reasons for failure of sequence

1. Haemolysis too rapid for liver to conjugate—Rh incompatibility, ABO incompatibility, sepsis, haematoma or other enclosed haemorrhage, inherited red cell defects; e.g. G6PD deficiency, congenital spherocytosis.

2. Insufficient albumen for binding because of presence of competitors; e.g. sulphonamides, salicylates, free fatty acids, or because binding reduced in acidosis.

3. Immaturity of glucuronyl transferase system in liver; e.g. in prematurity; or because of specific defect (Crigler-Najjan); or presence of pregnanediol in breast milk which inhibits system.

4. Mechanical blockage of bile preventing escape; e.g. in biliary atresia, certain infections causing hepatitis—rubella, herpes, cytomegalovirus.

5. Reabsorption of bile—overactive enterohepatic circulation.

Establishing cause of jaundice

Maternal history and tests would establish Rh. status. Normally part of ante-natal work up.

Occasionally unsuspected when mother fails to avail herself of facilities.

Family history of congenital haemolytic disease—look for spherocytosis or enzyme abnormalities.

Question regarding maternal drug intake—sulphas, aspirin.

Time of onset of jaundice indicative. At birth or within first 24 hours likely to be Rh incompatibility or infection. After first 24 hours—physiological normal.

Rare causes, galactosaemia in which galactose fails to be converted to glucose; hypothyroidism—thyroxine needed for glucuronide formation.

Laboratory tests

Red cell count. Percentage of reticulocytes—raised in haemolysis. White cell count for evidence of infection. Platelet count—reduced in infection. Red cell morphology for spherocytosis. Blood typing and cross matching with maternal blood. Haemagglutination tests for rubella, toxoplasmosis, CMV.

Bilirubin levels conjugated and unconjugated.

Blood gas studies to establish acidosis.

Urinary bilirubin and urobilinogen levels.

Blood protein levels especially albumen and albumen binding capacity.

Danger of jaundice

Conjugated bilirubin not dangerous in itself. Can be excreted freely in urine.

Unconjugated bilirubin not dangerous if below 20 mg/100 ml blood.

Up to this amount can be bound to serum albumen provided there are no competitors and sufficient albumin.

Danger from free, unbound, fat soluble bilirubin which crosses into lipid tissues of brain causing kernicterus.

Danger signs.

(1) Level of bilirubin exceeding 20 mg/100 ml blood.

(2) Low albumen binding capacity.

(3) Rapidly rising bilirubin levels in successive hourly samples even if well below 20 mg/100 ml.

Treatment

1. Phototherapy. Lowers unconjugated bilirubin levels in plasma. Useful when diagnosis of cause has been established

and danger of kernicterus absent; e.g. mild ABO incompatibility, secondary to sepsis, or when other methods are not possible. Also as an additional safeguard after exchange transfusion.

Daylight or 'blue light' fluorescent tubes which emit light of 300 to 600 millimicrons used. Child's eyes protected. Exposure to whole body for 24 hours continuously should lower serum bilirubin (unconjugated) by up to 8 mg/100 ml. Side effects noted include loose motions, skin rashes, pyrexia.

2. Phenobarbitone. Activates liver enzymes. Said to reduce unconjugated bilirubin. Controversial.

3. Exchange transfusion. Most used in Rh incompatibility, but useful in any condition when bilirubin levels rise too fast or high enough to cause kernicterus or in anaemia.

Fresh whole blood Group O, Rh negative used. 150 ml/kg body weight. Essential to monitor calcium levels, pH, potassium, temperature.

Kernicterus (Bilirubin encephalopathy)

Definition. Brain damage causing athetoid type of cerebral epilepsy, deafness for high frequencies and mental retardation.

Signs
Increasing jaundice, pyrexia, head retraction, opisthotonos, peculiar high pitched cry, twitching, convulsions, haemorrhage.

Cause
Destruction of brain cells by bilirubin which passes into lipid tissues when the albumen binding capacity for unconjugated bilirubin is exceeded. Before birth excess bilirubin excreted across placenta.

Treatment
Phototherapy. Exchange transfusion.

Haemolytic disease of newborn

Definition. Destruction of fetal red cells by antibodies transferred from maternal blood.

Cause
Immunisation of mother by antigens either from previous pregnancy or by blood transfusion.

Most commonly mother Rh (D)-negative, fetus Rh (D)-positive. Occasionally mother group O, fetus group A or B. Rarely mother A, fetus B or vice versa. Very rarely, specific antibodies present, Kell, Duffy, Lewis, Diego, etc.

Grades of severity

Mild. Moderate. Severe.

Mild—newborn is anaemic and jaundiced, but haemoglobin is above 12 g per cent and cord bilirubin below 4 mg per cent.

Moderate—icterus gravis. Infant pale at birth, haemoglobin below 12 g per cent. Umbilical cord stained yellow. Cord bilirubin above 4 mg per cent. Oedema and heart failure may be present.

Severe—hydrops fetalis. Gross oedema, ascites, pleural or pericardial effusion. Hepatosplenomegaly.

Prevention

Ante-natal grouping of mother's blood (and father's if mother is Rh negative) serves to warn of possible danger.

Injection of Rh antibody into mother within 72 hours of delivery (or abortion) destroys fetal red cells and prevents development of immunisation. This must be repeated after every pregnancy.

If immunisation has already occurred efforts made to minimize effect on fetus—induction of labour when it is judged that risks of prematurity are less than risk of hydrops developing. Intra-uterine transfusion of Group O Rh negative red blood cells into fetal peritoneal cavity may keep infant alive in utero for one or two weeks more—long enough to give it a fighting chance of survival.

Treatment

Clamp cord as soon as possible. Collect cord blood for haemoglobin and bilirubin levels. Transfuse to treat anaemia. Exchange transfuse to lower bilirubin and remove circulating antibody. Treat vigorously any other factors which reduce survival chances—immaturity, prematurity, low blood sugar, electrolyte upset, low serum calcium, acidosis.

Maturity

Almost all infants born between 37 and 40 weeks of gestation.

World Health Organisation defines an immature (premature) infant as one born before 37th week and a low birth weight (dysmature) infant as one weighing less than 2500 g.

Generally immature infants are also of low birth weight, but not necessarily so, while matured infants generally weigh more than 2500 g. Obviously gestational age and weight are insufficient guides to maturity by themselves.

Also it is important to distinguish between the immature infant and the mature, but low birth weight infant, because the problems are different for the two groups.

Immature infants, provided they get careful nursing in a protected environment will mature with the efflux of time, while dysmature infants are prone to aspiration pneumonia, have greater risk of bleeding, have poor temperature control, are prone to hypoglycaemia, become infected more readily.

Simple tests to distinguish immature from dysmature infants

1. *Glabellar tap*. Dysmature infant blinks.

   Immature does not before 32nd week.

2. *Heel to ear*. Dysmature—with difficulty.

   Immature—readily.

3. *Scarf sign*. (Wrapping arm round neck.)

   Dysmature—elbow does not reach midline.

   Immature—elbow passes readily to or beyond midline.

4. *Wrist and elbow flexion*. Dysmature—forced flexion brings hand or foot into contact with forearm or shin.

   Immature—full flexion impossible.

5. *Head rotation*. Dysmature—chin cannot be carried beyond acromion.

   Immature—chin can be rotated to or beyond acromion easily.

6. *Plantar creases*. Dysmature—sole covered with natural crease lines.

   Immature—smooth and creaseless.

7. *Crossed extensor reflex*. Stimulation of sole causes flexion of opposite hip and knee followed by extension, adduction and fanning of toes in dysmature.

   Immature—movements are indistinct and uncoordinated.

8. *Posture*. In prone position dysmature tucks knees under abdomen.

Immature lies flat with chest and abdomen in contact with cot and legs spread out.

9. *Moro reflex*. Dysmature responds to startle or falling manoeuvre by spreading arms wide then adducting them as if to embrace.

Immature—reflex absent or poorly coordinated.

Other indications of immature infant: head proportionally large; ear cartilages poorly developed; thin, deep red skin; lanugo marked all over; breast tissue absent; labia majora poorly developed revealing apparently overdeveloped labia minora and clitoris; poorly developed sucking and swallowing reflexes.

Care of immature and dysmature infants

Isolette or insul-cot incubators with control of humidity, temperature and oxygen ideal. Attendants reduced to minimum who should be freshly gowned, masked and washed before entering.

Oxygen given in sufficient concentration to prevent central cyanosis. For most, no added oxygen required. Indiscriminate use dangerous. Unnecessarily high concentration causes retrolental fibroplasia and pulmonary alveolar fibrosis.

Handling of small babies exhausts them. Generally no handling is permitted for up to 48 hours depending on birth weight.

Under 1360 g: 36 to 48 hours. 1360 to 2270 g: 24 hours, over 2270 g 12 to 24 hours.

Clothing—omitted in incubators. Light but warm wrappings in cot.

Feeding—glucose water for 24 hours either by bottle or by gavage tube graduating to breast milk or diluted formula so as to reach full calorie and fluid requirements by 10th day.

Specific problems dealt with as they arise. Close observations made and recorded regularly.

Congenital malformations

Incidence

Varies from country to country. Depends on facilities for collecting data, degree of sophistication of statistical services, motivation of reporters. Overall incidence of major malformations diagnosed at birth in Australia about 1·5 per cent live births. Approximately equal number come to light during first 12 months after birth. Similar figures in UK and USA.

Most common abnormalities

Anencephaly, hydrocephaly, talipes, cleft palate, spina bifida, cardiac anomalies, Down's syndrome.

Causes

Cause unknown in almost all cases. Known causes include some viral infections especially during 1st trimester—rubella, possibly influenza; irradiation—X-rays, radioactive substances; drugs—cytotoxics, anticoagulants, sulphonamides, antithyroid drugs, 19-norsteroids; anoxia; some inherited chromosomal defects.

Anencephaly

Definition. Failure to develop cranial vault and cerebrum.

Diagnosis. Suspected whenever hydramnios present. Confirmed by X-ray. Low maternal urinary oestriols.

Treatment. Induce labour at 34 weeks. Condition incompatible with life, but infant may survive up to 5 days.

Spina bifida

Definition. Failure to fuse of neural arches of one or more vertebrae so that cord and meninges not protected within tubular neural canal.

Grades. Minor—spina bifida occulta. Dimple in skin overlies defect in neural arch, but cord, meninges and spinal nerves unaffected.

Moderate—meningocoele. Dura mater lacking. Arachnoid and pia lie immediately beneath thin atrophic skin, but cord and nerves intact.

Severe—meningomyelocoele and myelocoele. Cord and spinal nerves involved.

In meningomyelocoele cord is covered by meninges, but skin deficient.

In myelocoele cord is a flattened sheet with no cover. Child paralysed, no sphincter control can develop.

In all grades there may be failure to develop of normal openings from 4th ventricle to allow escape of cerebrospinal fluid—Arnold-Chiari malformation—and hydrocephaly may develop.

Treatment. Cover defect with sterile material. Nurse face down. Meningocoele closed surgically within 24 hours. Severe forms sometimes closed similarly depending on state of infant. Most severer forms would succumb to anaesthetic anyway. Death from meningitis common.

Hydrocephaly

Definition. Distension of head with cerebrospinal fluid.

Cause. Failure to escape of CSF from ventricles to collection regions in subarachnoid space. Generally reason unknown. Occasionally toxoplasma infection.

Onset. May be ante-natal. Causes difficulties in delivery. Vertex presenting may not engage. Breech presenting may result in impaction of aftercoming head.

May be post-natally. Weekly measurement of head circumference reveals increase greater than 0·6 cm. Bulging fontanelles at birth suspicious.

Treatment. Gross hydrocephaly at birth not treated. Insertion of bypass or shunt from lateral ventricle to neck vein or right atrium worthwhile if head size not too altered at birth.

Microcephaly

Whole head and brain smaller than normal. Child may survive but mental retardation severe.

Craniostenosis

One or more sutures close prematurely preventing normal coordinated growth of cranium. Head mis-shaped depending on which suture is closed. Surgical splitting of affected suture allows normal expansion and prevents mental retardation.

Cleft lip and cleft palate

Definition. Failure to fuse of bones and overlying skin or mucous membranes. In embryo roof of mouth, anterior gums and upper lip form during second month from 2 palatine processes, 2 maxillary processes and median nasal process. Any one or more of these may fail to reach its opposite number. Defects occur from mere indentation, to complete absence of front of upper lip, incisor part of gum and roof of mouth. Most common form is unilateral lip cleft only—1st week of life. Bilateral— about 3 months.

Cleft palate about one year, before speech habits develop.

Severe forms with large deficit may need dental plates to pull edges of deficit closer together before surgery undertaken.

Talipes

Definition. Mal-alignment of foot with leg. Many terms applied depending on position of foot—equino varus, calcaneo valgus.

Treatment. Forced correction of position and maintenance of correction with strapping, splints or splints or plaster. Should be done on 1st day of birth.

Congenital dislocation of hip

Definition. Flattening of acetabulum which allows developing head of femur to lie outside its cup against ilium.

Diagnosis. Ortolani's test (see page 124). X-ray.

Treatment. Affected limb (often bilateral) held in flexion and abduction by splint or plaster for 8 to 12 weeks. This keeps head of femur against acetabulum and allows it to develop into proper cup.

If diagnosis missed at birth chances of correction by simple means diminish rapidly. At 2 years of age very little hope of cure.

Down's syndrome (Mongol)

Definition. Trisomy 21; i.e. extra piece of chromosome material making 47 chromosomes instead of normal 46.

Occurrence. Overall 1 in 1000 births, but incidence rises steeply with age of mother. Over 45 incidence is 3 per cent.

Recognition. Eyes slanting. Epicanthic folds. Ears small, square and lacking cartilage. Down-turned corners to mouth. Narrow pointed tongue often protruding. Skin dry and scaly. Fingers short, all of similar length. Little finger curved laterally. Big toe widely separated. Single palmar crease. General hypotonia. Not all these features need be present.

Diagnosis. Chromosome studies.

Treatment. Nil. Explain nature of condition to both parents.

Achondroplasia

Definition. Defect of cartilage affecting humeri and femora markedly, but all long bones to some extent. Cause unknown.

Incidence. 1 in 10 000 births.

Severity. Varies. Most grow to adulthood without mental defect. No treatment.

Digestive tract anomalies

Oesophageal atresia

Definition. Failure of continuity of oesophagus, with or without fistula connecting trachea. Cause unknown.

Diagnosis. Suspect in hydramnios. Attempt to pass No. 8 or 9 English gauge Jaques rubber catheter before any feed given. Copious frothy mucous suspicious. X-ray with oily contrast medium confirms.

Treatment. Surgical correction possible in 70 per cent. Multiple atresias throughout bowel sometimes present.

Duodenal atresia

Definition. Failure of continuity of lumen of duodenum.

Diagnosis. Suspect if persistent bile stained vomiting occurs. Confirmed by barium meal.

Treatment. Surgical correction.

Pyloric stenosis

Definition. Thickening and spasm of pyloric sphincter.

Diagnosis. Suspect if otherwise healthy child starts projectile vomiting in 2nd to 3rd week.

More common in males. Mass 2 cm in diameter felt in right upper quadrant of abdomen. Visible peristalsis waves seen in epigastrium.

Treatment. Lesser degrees respond to antispasmodics 15 to 20 minutes before feeds, dicyclomine (Merbentyl) 2·5 mg; atropine methonitrate (Eumydrin) 2 drops of 0·6 per cent alcoholic solution; pipenzolate bromide (Piptal) 2 mg.

Surgical correction—Ramstedt's operation—hypertrophic sphincter split longitudinally down to mucous membrane.

Malrotation

Definition. Persistence of early embryonic form of gut development. Colon short and occupies left lower portion of abdomen, caecum lies in front of right kidney, duodenum spirally coiled. Lack of attachment of mesentery.

Diagnosis. Usually unsuspected until intestinal obstruction occurs. Barium meal confirms. Volvulus common.

Treatment. Surgical relief of intestinal obstruction, correction of volvulus, fixation of bowel.

Umbilical hernia

Definition. Persistence of a hole through midline at umbilicus through which peritoneum, omentum, gut may protrude to lie under skin.

Diagnosis. Simple palpation.

Treatment. Observe over following 18 months. Most close spontaneously by this age. If still patent, surgical closure to prevent strangulation.

Imperforate anus

Definition. Failure to develop an opening between rectum and exterior.

Degrees: Minor. Persistence of anal membrane only.
Major. Colon ends blind above pelvic floor.

Diagnosis. By post-natal inspection.

Treatment. Surgical correction in minor degrees in which anal sphincter present. Colostomy in major degrees.

Cardiac anomalies

Incidence: 0·6 per cent of live births.

Many cardiac anomalies incompatible with life. Commonly occurring anomalies amenable to correction: Patent ductus arteriosus. Septal defects. Tetralogy of Fallot. Coarctation of aorta.

Paten ductus arteriosus

Definition. Persistence of communication between arch of aorta and bifurcation of right and left pulmonary arteries.

Diagnosis. Systolic and diastolic murmurs—continuous 'machinery' murmur—best heard over 2nd to 3rd left intercostal space with wide transmission, wide pulse pressure, enlarged left atrium and ventricle, X-ray shows increased pulmonary vascular markings and pulsatile pulmonary arteries.

Treatment. Surgical division and ligation of ductus as soon as possible in otherwise healthy infant.

In all cardiac abnormalities high risk of bacterial endocarditis exists.

Septal defects
1. Atrial
2. Ventricular.

Atrial septal defect

Definition. Persistence of embryonic foramen into postnatal life.

Diagnosis. Systolic murmur loudest over 2nd left interspace transmitted to apex. Wide, fixed splitting of second sound. X-ray shows enlargement of right side of heart. Flow studies confirm diagnosis.

Treatment. Surgical closure.

Ventricular septal defect

Definition. Congenital failure of interventricular septum to meet right atrioventricular cushion. Hole may be small or large. If small no signs or symptoms may arise.

Diagnosis. Harsh systolic murmur often with palpable thrill over 3rd left space. X-ray may show left ventricular enlargement, increased pulmonary vascular markings. Diagnosis confirmed by flow studies.

Treatment. Depends on severity of left to right shunting. Closure attempted in serious cases at 4 to 5 years of age. Bacterial endocarditis guarded against with penicillin prophylaxis.

Tetralogy of Fallot

Definition. Four features: (1) Pulmonary stenosis; (2) Ventricular septal defect; (3) Aorta overrides septal defect; (4) Patent ductus arteriosus.

Diagnosis. Systolic murmur loudest at lower left sternal edge. Single second sound. X-ray may show 'boot-shaped' heart. ECG shows left ventricular hypertrophy. Cyanosis variable depending on readiness with which aorto-pulmonary shunting occurs via ductus arteriosus. As ductus closes cyanosis becomes severe.

Treatment. If cyanosis severe—arterio-pulmonary anastomosis. Later, repair of septum and of pulmonsry stenosis may be possible.

Coarctation of aorta

Definition. Constriction of aorta just beyond ductus arteriosus.

Diagnosis. Systolic murmur loudest at left infraclaviculr region radiating to midline posteriorly. Femoral pulses less marked and delayed after radial pulses. Arterial pressure greater in arms than legs. Confirmation from flow studies.

Treatment. Resection and anastomosis at about 6 months.

Uro-genital anomalies

Clitoral enlargement

Progestin therapy during pregnancy causes tendency towards masculinization which regresses in most cases. Occasionally, plastic surgery needed.

In adreno-genital syndrome increased formation of ACTH results from low blood levels of cortisone. High ACTH levels overstimulates production of androgen causing masculinization of female organs—clitoral enlargement and fusion of labia.

Diagnosis. Careful examination of genitalia essential. Often sex equivocal by inspection.

Could be boy with bilateral undescended testes and hypospadias. Chromosome studies and laparotomy may be needed.

Treatment. Check adrenal function and electrolytes. Often lack of aldosterone cause rapidly fatal loss of sodium and retention of potassium. Correction of genital anomalies not urgent.

Hypospadias

Definition. Urinary meatus opens other than at tip of penis.

Treatment. Depends on site of opening.

Minor malplacement under glans common and needs no correction.

May be associated with chordee—curvature of penis due to fibrous band. Correction by excision of band. Prepuce may be useful for skin graft or formation of urethra to bring meatus to tip of penis.

Low penile and scrotal hypospadias rare. Plastic operations needed.

Ectopic testes

Definition. Descent of testes into scrotum arrested.

Diagnosis. One (most commonly) or both testes absent from scrotum. May be possible to palpate in inguinal region.

Treatment. Orchidopexy before ten years of age.

Ectopia vesicae

Definition. Lower part of abdominal wall covered with transitional epithelium which merges with normal skin. Ureteric orifices open on to this area.

Treatment. Plastic surgery to close skin defect. Transplantation of ureters into 'false bladder' fashioned from isolated loop of ileum or piece of colon.

Minor disorders

Diarrhoea

Breast fed neonates usually pass meconium on days 1 and 2 then soft greeny-gold motions three or four times daily for 5 to 6 weeks. More frequent passage especially if very moist, constitutes diarrhoea.

Causes. 1. Dietary imbalance. 2. Infection. 3. Associated with other disease; e.g. carbohydrate intolerance, cystic fibrosis, congenital adrenal hyperplasia.

Dietary imbalance

Most likely to arise in bottle fed babies. Too dilute feeds, excessive quantity, indigestible contents. Proprietary brands which are 'humanized' give least trouble. Cows milk—most.

Occasionally lactose intolerance is cause.

Treatment—investigate feeding and adjust.

Infection

Often establistment of cause not achieved. Bacteria and viruses difficult to isolate even in epidemics. Gastro-enteritis not uncommon in spite of stringent precautions.

Treatment—Fluid replacement with oral glucose fluids if tolerable, otherwise IV.

Monitor electrolyte twice daily.

Culture stools. Isolate affected infants. If organism can be demonstrated, appropriate antibiotic may be given, but fluid and electrolyte replacement considered sufficient.

Other diseases. When diarrhoea fails to improve within few days further investigation instituted.

Constipation

Uncommon in newborn.

Rare causes. Mucoviscidosis (cystic fibrosis), Hirschsprung's disease (infantile megacolon). Common cause in later days—inadequate fluid intake.

Mucoviscidosis

Definition. Generalised malformation of exocrine glands affecting those making sweat, mucus, pancreatic secretions, saliva, tears.

Signs and symptoms. Meconium ileus present at birth. Thick, clay-like meconium. Marked increase in chloride content of sweat. Assay of pancreatic fluid shows markedly decreased enzymes. Early onset of respiratory infections, pulmonary fibrosis, hepatic fibrosis.

Treatment. Early recognition. Nurse in Isolette with high humidity. Add pancreatic enzymes to feeds. Reduce fat and increase protein in feeds. Antibiotics according to sensitivity tests early in infections. Immunise early against pertussis. Replace sodium chloride by adding salt to feeds.

Hirschsprung's disease

Definition. Absence of myenteric plexus and hence incoordination of peristalsis in a section of colon, leading to gross distension of colon proximally. Site of absence commonly recto-sigmoid.

Signs. Complete constipation. Progressive abdominal distension.

Diagnosis. X-ray shows distended loops of small and large intestine ending abruptly at site of aganglionic section.

Rectal biopsy must include muscularis mucosa to reveal aganglionic state.

Treatment. Early resection of aganglionic section and anastomosis prevents gross megacolon. Occasionally colostomy necessary.

Skin colour changes and birth marks

During delivery cyanosis may be severe. After initial breath skin becomes uniformly pink or frankly red. Hands and feet may remain pale for few hours.

Superficial angiomata common at birth. Bright red spots or areas. May grow rapidly for six months then regress spontaneously.

Capillary haemangiomata do not blanch on pressure. Often violet or purple. Smaller ones may respond to plastic surgery. Most often have to be accepted. Occasionally associated with arterio-venous anomalies of meninges. Sturge-Weber syndrome—epileptiform convulsions.

Cyanosis. Vasomotor instability causes transient cyanosis in newborn. Persistent cyanosis always serious and cause should be sought—respiratory, cardiac, haemorrhage, sepsis, metabolic.

Petechiae. Capillary haemorrhage causing dark spots in mucous membranes and skin. Causes include infections, blood disorders causing clotting defects especially thrombocytopaenia, maternal intake of some drugs which depress platelet formation.

Following prolonged or difficult birth a few petechiae may be found round the head, which soon fade.

Vomit scalding. Delicate skin of newborn easily damaged by gastric acid. Should be wiped away and soiled clothing removed.

Breast engorgement. Common in boys and girls. Due to maternal hormone withdrawal. May persist, rarely for 6-12 months. No treatment, provided infection excluded.

11. Maternal and Perinatal Statistics

Maternal Mortality

Definition. Deaths due to pregnancy and childbirth. Usually expressed as a rate—number of deaths per 1000 registered births, live and still, during any year.

Collection of data
In almost all countries notification of births and deaths compulsory. An informant, usually a relative, must register the fact of death on receipt of certificate signed by doctor or other qualified person. In most countries other relevant facts also recorded—WHO recommendations being adopted slowly.

Comparative figures
Maternal mortality fallen spectacularly since 1930. Rate in Western countries in 1930 between 40 and 50. Now rate between 0·2 and 0·3. Usual now to quote actual number of deaths in a country rather than rate.

Former causes of death
Before 1930, major causes of maternal mortality in UK—sepsis 25 per cent. Toxaemia (pre-eclampsia and eclampsia) 20 per cent. Haemorrhage 12 per cent. Abortion 18 per cent. Thrombo-embolism 7 per cent.

Present causes of death
In 1966, causes were—abortion 24 per cent, toxaemia 17 per cent, haemorrhage 12 per cent, thrombo-embolism 5 per cent, sepsis 4 per cent.

Research
Most countries now have committees to examine causes of maternal mortality and make recommendations for prevention. Improvements due to introduction of antibiotics, blood transfusion services, improvements in maternity hospitals and obstetric care, higher standard of living generally.

National Health and Medical Research Council of Australia

sets up expert committee to examine causes of maternal mortality over 3 yearly periods. This committee found that during triennium 1967–69 43 per cent of deaths were avoidable; e.g. those due to haemorrhage, many due to pre-eclampsia and eclampsia, infection. Early recognition of possibility of danger essential.

Vital statistics

Definition
Numerical data concerned with the life and health of individuals in society.

Necessary to:
1. Assess present population quantity + quality
2. Plan for future needs e.g. schools, houses, hospitals, social services, employment, transport etc.
3. Compare efficiency of services in different areas and countries
4. Recognize trends—adverse or otherwise.

Information from:

1. The census. Conducted every 10 years since 1801 by Registrar Generals Office (Mini-census of 10 per cent of the population every 5 years). Questionaire sent to every household results in information on
   a. Population quantity—total number of people
   b. Population quality—age, sex, structure, social status (occupation) etc.

2. Notification of births—ALL live and stillbirths
Compulsory since 1915
TO Area Medical Officer.
BY Midwife or someone else present AT or WITHIN 6 hours of birth.
WITHIN 36 hours.
WHY? (i) Vital Statistics—including incidence of prematurity, congenital abnormality; (ii) To alert Area Health Authority re—new baby to be cared for—i.e. follow up visit by Health Visitor, Observation register; (iii) To inform local Registrars office (double check to ensure registration).

3. Registration of Births—ALL live and stillbirths

Compulsory since 1926

TO Local Registrar.

BY Parent(s) or someone else present at the birth i.e. Midwife WITHIN 42 days.

WHY? (i) Vital Statistics; (ii) To issue a) Birth certificate + N.H.S. card IF live. b) Disposal certificate. IF stillbirth; (iii) To check notification.

4. Registration of Deaths

TO Local Registrar.

BY Relatives.

WITHIN 5 days.

WHY? (i) Vital statistics. (ii) To issue Disposal Certificate.

Registrar general

Collects, collates and publishes results in annual statistical review.

Vital statistics

Expressed as RATES per 1000 total population per year. OR per 1000 of a specific population group per year.

1. Birth rate. Number of live births per 1000 population per year.

2. Stillbirth rate. Number of stillbirths per 1000 total births per year.

Definition of stillbirth—A baby who, after being completely expelled from the birth canal after 28th week of pregnancy does not breath or show any other signs of life.

3. Perinatal mortality rate. Number of stillbirths PLUS deaths in the first week of life per 1000 total births per year.

Details in British Births 1970 Volume I*.

4. Neonatal mortality rate. Number of deaths in the first month of life per 1000 live births per year.

5. Infant mortality rate. Number of deaths in the first year of life per 1000 live births per year.

6. Maternal mortality rate. Number of deaths associated with pregnancy and childbirth per 1000 total births per year.

Report on Confidential Enquiries into Maternal Deaths in England & Wales gives details of major causes.

---

* A survey by National Birthday Trust Fund and Royal College of Obstetricians and Gynaecologists.

In 1970 to 72:
1. Abortion
2. Pulmonary Embolism
3. Toxaemia (Eclampsia and pre-eclampsia)
4. Ectopic pregnancy
5. Sepsis (excluding abortion)

7. *Abortion*. Any interruption of pregnancy before the 28th week with dead fetus.

Perinatal morbidity and mortality

Definitions (WHO recommendations.)

Fetal death. Death occurring before complete expulsion or extraction from mother of product of conception regardless of duration of pregnancy.

This definition embraces what were formerly called stillbirths, abortions and miscarriages.

Perinatal period. From 28th week to 7th day of life.

Abortion. Any interruption of pregnancy before 28th week with dead fetus.

Live birth. Any product of conception which, after complete separation from its mother, breathes or shows any evidence of life, irrespective of duration of pregnancy.

Perinatal mortality. This refers to deaths occurring between 28th week and 7th day of life.

Neonatal deaths. Those occurring up to 28 days after birth.

Stillbirth: WHO recommends abandonment of the term 'stillbirth.' Still commonly used.

Definition: Stillborn child is one born after 20th week of gestation, which shows no heartbeat, respiration or movement at any time after delivery.

Causes

Antepartum deaths closely related to eclampsia, pre-eclampsia and antepartum haemorrhage.

Intrapartum deaths related to degree of skill in diagnosing complications and method of delivery especially in malposition.

Postpartum deaths related to prematurity and low birth weight, malformations and infections.

Actual causes of death are hypoxia, malformation, prematurity, infection, intracranial haemorrhage, erythroblastosis.

Time of neonatal deaths
60 per cent in first 24 hours and two thirds of those within first 6 hours; 24 per cent during 2nd and 3rd days; 7·5 per cent during 4th to 7th days; 9·5 per cent during 2nd to 4th weeks.

Other contributory factors
Small mother—less than 150 cm (5ft); parity; risk increases for fourth child and upwards; maternal age, risk increases rapidly after 30 years; previous history of abnormal pregnancy; birth weight—risk greater below 2500 g.

12. Family Planning

Infertility

Inability to conceive though apparently normal.

Causes

Male — Lack of sufficient viable spermatozoa due to: deficiency of FSH or ICSH, aspermia, failure of spermatozoa to develop normally, occlusion of vasa deferentia.

Other male causes when sperm are normal—impotence, ignorance, premature ejaculation.

Female—Tubal obstruction, excessive acidity of vagina, anovulatory cycles, immunological destruction of sperm, endometrial deficiency, presence of fibroma, carcinoma, or hyperprolactinaemia.

Investigations

Detailed questioning of both partners may reveal faulty sex techniques, ignorance, impotence. Relative aspermia may result from too frequent intercourse.

Semen analysis. Semen collected into a special condom during intercourse. Condom must be free of spermicidal lubricant. Many laboratories examine semen collected by masturbation. Normal values are up to 5 ml volume with 50 to 150 million sperms per ml, 80 per cent fully motile and less than 25 per cent of abnormal forms. Sterility if less than 20 million per ml, more than 20 per cent immotile or more than 40 per cent abnormal.

Testicular biopsy may reveal pathology of testis.

Hühner's test performed when sperm count and sperm motility normal. Sperm's collected from vagina by aspiration immediately after intercourse. Motility of less than 75 per cent indicates immunological rejection of sperm or too high acid medium.

Examination of cervical mucus. At ovulation character of mucus alters. Mucin aggregates into long strands which allow free passage of sperms. Also allows mucus to be drawn out into thread up to 10 cm long without breaking (Spinnbarkeit). At other times mucus thick, viscid, impenetrable.

Ovulation tests. At ovulation corpus luteum develops and progesterone is produced. Changes brought about by progesterone taken as evidence that ovulation has occurred; e.g. endometrium shows secretory pattern, vaginal wall desquamates small, round, granular cells, basal body temperature rises $0.5°C$, ferning of cervical mucus fails to occur.

Direct measurement of oestrogen, progesterone. FSH and LH now performed by immuno-assay on blood or urine.

Tests of tubal patency. Rubins test. Carbon dioxide blown through tube fitted tightly into cervix. Manometer measures pressure of gas within uterus and tubes. At 200 mmHg stethoscope placed over left and right iliac fossae may detect hiss of escaping gas through fimbriae of each tube. If pressure stays at 200 mmHg when gas turned off both tubes are blocked. If pressure rapidly falls off at least one tube is patent.

Hysterosalpingography more informative than Rubins test. Introduction of radio opaque material shows whether tubes are patent and reveals abnormalities of uterus if shape of cavity altered.

Curettings of endometrium reveal presence of cancer cells, tuberculosis, fibromata, fibrosis.

Treatment of infertility depends on revealed causative factors if any. Often no abnormality detected. Advice then needed to ensure highest chance of conception—reduction of frequency of intercourse to ensure high sperm counts, intercourse soon after ovulation detected by careful temperature recordings. Following intercourse dorsal posture maintained for two hours with buttocks or foot of bed elevated to facilitate sperm retention.

Anovulation may have pituitary or ovarian causes. Correction of these not always possible, but replacement therapy may stimulate ovulation. Human pituitary gonadotrophin injected on alternate days for 14 days. Human chorionic gonadotrophin on twelfth days acts like LH and ovulation usually occurs.

Prolactin normally secreted during pregnancy and lactation. Suppresses ovulation and menstruation.

Inappropriate secretion causes infertility in women and hypogonadism in men. Treatment with bromocriptine reduces secretion of prolactin and allows other pituitary hormones to work. Dosage: 5–7·5 mg daily.

Clomiphene increases secretion of normal FSH. 50 mg orally for five days followed by ovulation in five days.

Tubal obstruction sometimes overcome by incision through obstruction and sewing edges open—salpingostomy. Ovaries inspected at same time, adhesions freed, tumours removed. Excision of cornual obstruction and re-implantation of tubes or implantation of ovary into wall of uterus sometimes tried.

Contraception

Methods to prevent pregnancy by preventing conception, or implantation.

Methods to keep sperm from ova:
1. Coitus interruptus
2. Condom
3. Vaginal diaphragm
4. Minipill. (Progestogen only)
5. Rhythm method
6. Tubal ligation.

Methods to destroy sperm:
1. Vaginal douche
2. Spermicidal creams and foams
3. Male pill
4. Vasectomy.

Methods to suppress ovulation:
1. Contraceptive pill

Methods to prevent implantation:
1. Progestogens
2. Intra-uterine device.

Coitus interruptus. Penis withdrawn just before male climax. High failure rate. Great dissatisfaction psychologically and physiologically.

Condom. Thin rubber sheath placed over penis. Suitable lubricant, often spermicidal, renders it almost undetectable during coitus. Satisfactory, but interrupts spontaneity. May become dislodged. May have holes in it if stored too long.

Vaginal diaphragm. Shallow rubber cup with spring loaded

circumferential rim. Extends from posterior fornix to behind symphysis pubis. Spermicidal jelly placed in cup before insertion so that cervix immersed. Disadvantages same as condom—may dislodge, may have holes.

'Minipill'. Progestogen only. Norethisterone 0·35 mg. Alters consistency of cervical mucus making it difficult for sperm to penetrate. No effect on ovulation. Higher failure rate than other contraceptive pills—4 failures per 100 women-years; i.e. if 100 women use minipill as sole means of contraception for one year, 4 become pregnant. Alternatively, if a woman uses minipill solely she will become pregnant once in 25 years.

Useful method for females in danger of thrombosis, who are lactating or who may have reached climacteric, but do not want the risk of pregnancy until sure.

Rhythm method. Abstinence from coitus before, during and after ovulation. Time of ovulation established by carefully kept temperature charts extending over several cycles. Temperature taken at same time every day, using same thermometer and same route, preferably rectal or vaginal. Rise in basal temperature is small—0·5 to 0·75°C only. Careless recording can easily miss it. Once regular pattern established coitus stops from 3 days before expected day of ovulation to 4 days after actual day as determined from temperature.

Method is only one sanctioned by R.C. prelate.

Disadvantages—ovulation may occur early, sperm may remain active for 48 hours causing high failure rate.

Tubal ligation. (See page 105.) Permanent barrier to sperm. Experiments proceeding to make tubal interference a reversible process, but poor results so far.

Vaginal douche. Effective in cleaning out vagina if carried out within seconds of coitus. Spermicidal solutions used— vinegar, quinine, lead acetate. However, method quite ineffective in removing sperm already through cervix. If satisfactory orgasm occurs uterus exerts powerful suction effect which draws semen through cervix.

Spermicidal creams. Many substances very effective in rendering sperm immobile in laboratory, but mixing semen with cream inside vagina far from effective especially if male climax and female orgasm occur simultaneously and semen immediately aspirated. Best used inside condom or diaphragm.

Male 'pill'. Experiments proceeding to supress spermatogenesis without interfering with production of testosterone. Not yet ready for use on humans.

Vasectomy. Removal of sections of vasa deferentia and ligation performed through small incisions in scrotum. Highly successful form of contraception. Irreversible, hence recipient must be sure he will not wish to father more children.

Contraceptive pill. Many combinations of oestrogens and progestins. All work by indirectly suppressing ovulation. Oestrogens suppress FSH releasing factor hence insufficient FSH released from anterior pituitary, hence follicles fail to mature, hence ovulation does not occur.

Oestrogen itself cannot be given orally because of destruction by gastric juice. Hence synthetically altered oestrogens used—ethinyloestradiol or mestranol 30 to 100 mg.

Progestogens inhibit LH releasing factor, inhibit cervical mucus production, inhibit tubal transport, encourage atypical endometrium hostile to fertilized ovum. Nine different progestogens in use for oral contraceptives. Various combinations manufactured by different firms. Very little real difference between them.

Most common type of pill—combination pill—oestrogen and progestogen together for 21 days starting day 1 of menstruation, then nothing for 7 days (or sugar pill for 7 days). Bleeding occurs sometime during these 7 days. Not normal menstruation. Usually diminished in quantity and duration. Free from pain. Predictable. Tends to follow same pattern exactly in every cycle.

Sequential pill supplies oestrogen only for 15 days then oestrogen plus progestogen for 5 days. Resembles normal physiological pattern of hormone secretion. Used when continuous progestogens produce side effects attributable to progesterone.

Complications. Many side-effects blamed on oral contraceptives without adequate proof—depression, increased libido, decreased libido, fatigue. Some side effects proved; e.g. fluid retention and increase in appetite leading to weight gain; occasionally increased hirsutism on high progestogen pill; nausea from high oestrogen pill; chloasma; alteration of cholesterol and triglyceride levels.

Occasionally persistent side effects occur e.g. breast tenderness, and break through bleeding (BTB). Latter controlled by changing formulation. BTB occuring early in cycle, during first 7–10 days responds to increased oestrogens, that occurring in latter half, 10–24 days, to increased progestagen.

Acne can be a nuisance due to sensitivity to some progestogens. Changing to pill with moderate oestrogen and low progestogen may improve condition.

Contra-indications to Pill

Epilepsy. Likelihood of fits increased. Can be off-set by increasing phenytoin or phenobaritone.

Age over 35. Other methods advised.

Lactation. Oestrogen suppresses lactation. Progestogen only pill is suitable.

Thrombosis. Any history of thrombosis is absolute contra-indication.

Migraine. Care should be taken that pill does not precipitate headaches. Lowest available dosage recommended.

Antibiotics. Rifampicin in treatment of tuberculosis is contraindication. Other antibiotics may reduce absorption and alternative contraception advised until course finished.

Hypertension. Preferably use alternative means of contraception.

Most important complication, thrombosis, especially when susceptibility increased; e.g. in clotting defect, liver disease, diabetes and smoking especially.

Also, following history of irregular and scanty periods before starting oral contraceptives, occasional patient found to be anovulatory on cessation—post-pill infertility.

Carcinoma of breast and uterus not increased among Pill takers. Benign adenoma of liver increased in long term use, but still a very rare tumour. Incidence of cancer of ovary reduced among Pill users.

Benefits of contraceptive pill

Marked reduction of menorrhagia. Reduced incidence of breast fibroplasia. Little or no dysmenorrhoea. Reduction in iron deficiency anaemia. Less premenstrual tension. Fewer incidences of ovarian cyst formation.

Termination of pregnancy

(See page 42) Very few countries encourage abortion as a means of family limitation. However, laws in many countries interpreted more leniently than hitherto and legal action rarely taken where abortion carried out by legally registered medical practitioner for genuine health reasons which include psychiatric danger to mother if pregnancy continues.

Little danger to woman if carried out in first trimester. However, risks incurred—sepsis, Rh. immunisation, haemorrhage, shock. Second trimester abortions carry greater maternal risk depending on method used. Intra-amniotic infusion of hypertonic saline—absorption causing convulsions, cerebral infarction; IV oxytocin—hypertension.

13. Anatomy and Physiology

The Bony Pelvis

Ring of bones supporting abdominal organs, but allowing passage to exterior.

Components
Right and left innominate laterally and anteriorly, sacrum and coccyx posteriorly. Innominate bones made up of pubic bones united by ligamentous joint anteriorly, ischium inferiorly, ilium forming broad shelf superiorly.

Posteriorly, five sacral vertebrae fused into one mass, the sacrum, unite with right and left ilia at sacro-iliac joints.

Coccyx, four tiny vertebrae attached to sacrum inferiorly. Forms anchorage for midline of muscles forming pelvic diaphragm.

Cavity of pelvis: Pelvic cavity divided into 'true' and 'false' portions by roughly circular edge of bone formed by body of first sacral vertebra (sacral promontory), ilio-pectineal line and eminence, and the arcuate line of ilium and pubis. Above line is 'false' pelvis—mainly supportive, below is 'true' pelvis in which lies bladder, uterus, tubes, ovaries, rectum.

True pelvis forms basin-like structure. Open upper part of basin communicates freely with abdominal cavity. Lower part of basin closed by pelvic floor of muscle. Pelvic organs attached to pelvic floor which is pierced by urethra, vagina and anal canal. Peritoneum lining abdominal cavity continues into pelvic cavity and forms supporting ligaments. Peritoneum draped over uterus and tubes forms broad ligament and extends laterally to divide true pelvis into anterior and posterior portions. Anterior portion occupied by bladder. Peritoneum dips down between bladder and uterus, vesico-uterine pouch, and may extend to lie between urethra and vagina. Posterior portion occupied by rectum. Similarly, peritoneum dips down uterus and rectum to form utero-rectal pouch or pouch of Douglas. May extend to lie between vagina and anterior rectal wall.

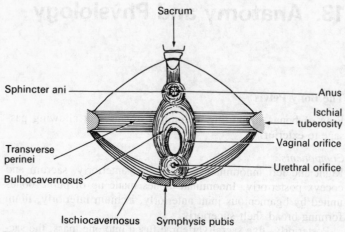

Fig. 13.1 Diagram looking into the pelvis to illustrate the superficial muscles of the pelvic floor.

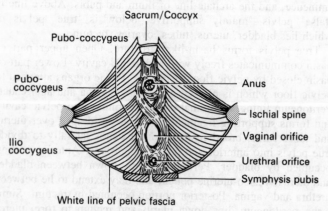

Fig. 13.2 Diagram looking into the pelvis to illustrate the (levator ani) deep muscles of the pelvic floor.

Pelvic inlet

Opening into true pelvis, usually called the 'inlet' or 'brim'. Most commonly almost circular. Lateral diameter 12·7 to 14 cm, anteroposterior diameter 10·8 to 11·4 cm. Great variation. Types: Gynaecoid—almost circular; Anthropoid—narrower laterally; Android—heart shaped, wider posteriorly. Platypelloid—oval, wider laterally.

Pelvic cavity

Curves forward so that posterior sacral wall is longer than anterior pubic wall. Usually almost circular measuring 11·4 to 12·7 cm in all diameters.

Pelvic outlet

Limited by sub-pubic angle anteriorly, spines of ischia laterally, and sacro-coccyx posteriorly. Ligaments extend between these points—sacrospinous ligament easily palpable vaginally forms valuable landmark. Ligaments make outlet diamond shaped.

Subpubic angle ideally greater than 90° as in gynaecoid and platypelloid pelves.

Pelvic floor

Mainly of muscle divided into deep or internal layer and superficial or external layer.

Deep layer: Levator ani, right and left, extend from ligament between ischial spine and pubis to sacrum. Hammock like. Meet in mid-line. Thicken and criss-cross in mid-line, to form voluntary sphincters round urethra, vagina and anal canal. Posteriorly muscular floor completed by coccygeus muscles. Superficial layer: Perineal muscles. Transverse perinei extend laterally from perineum to tuberosity of ischium. Bulbocavernosus extend form perineum one on each side of vagina to join above clitoris. Ischio cavernosus extend from ramus of ischium on each side of clitoris to tuberosity of ischium. These muscles easily damaged by tearing during delivery or by episiotomy.

Nerves and vessels

Rich nerve supply to genital region. Sympathetic sensory from uterus pass to lower thoracic spinal segments. Somatic sensory from vagina, clitoris, labia, perineum transmitted via inferior rectal, perineal and dorsal nerve of clitoris through sacral plexus to sacral segments 2, 3 and 4. Skin sensations transmitted through ilio-inguinal and genito-femoral nerves via lumbar plexus and lumbar segments 1 to 5 and sacral 1.

Blood vessels derived from internal iliac arteries via uterine and vaginal branches. Also from ovarian arteries derived from aorta directly. These anastomose within broad ligament. Whole network greatly expanded and augmented during pregnancy.

External genitalia supplied by internal iliac artery which terminates as internal pudendal artery to labia, clitoris, urethra, perineum.

Venous drainage follows arteries and enters internal iliac vessels. Also ovarian veins, left into left renal vein, right into inferior vena cava.

Lymphatic drainage from body of uterus, fallopian tubes and ovaries pass directly into para-aortic nodes. From cervix three routes pass to (1) external iliac nodes, (2) internal iliac nodes, (3) backwards to sacral nodes.

A few lymphatics accompany round ligament along inguinal canal and hence to inguinal nodes.

Vaginal lymphatics unite with those of cervix, body of uterus and rectal. Those of labia, clitoris, perineum drain via superficial inguinal nodes.

Vulva

Definition. Those parts of external genitalia which can be seen. Comprise labia majora, labia minora, clitoris, vaginal orifice.

Labia majora
Two fatty pads of tissue extending from mons pubis overlying symphysis pubis anteriorly passing one on each side of vaginal orifice to perineum.

Labia minora
Lie within labia majora. Thin folds of skin uniting posteriorly to form fourchette. Anteriorly labia minora divide to form folds enclosing the clitoris. Anterior folds form prepuce of clitoris.

Clitoris
Highly sensitive structure analogous to penis. Lies 2 cm anterior to urethral orifice.

Vaginal orifice or introitus

Surrounded by tags of skin of former hymen—carunculae myrtiformes. Useful guideline during repair of episiotomy to line up sides of incision correctly.

Bartolins glands

Lie in posterior part of labia majora. Secrete a lubricant.

Perineum

Region between fourchette and anus. Overlies perineal body, a wedge shaped structure of fibrous tissue forming anchorage for perineal muscles.

Vagina

Tubular structure, highly distensible, but normally collapsed, extending from vestibule to cervix. Cervix protrudes into upper anterior part of vault and demarcates 4 arches or fornices—anterior, posterior, right and left lateral.

Relationships

Superior—uterus and adnexae;
Anterior—urethra and posterior wall of bladder;
Posterior—rectum and perineal body.

Pouch of Douglas intervenes between rectum and vagina to variable extent posteriorly. Entry to peritoneal cavity afforded through posterior fornix. Ureters approach closely to lateral fornices.

Structure

Inner lining of stratified epithelium similar to skin, but without stratum corneum. Epithelium reflected onto cervix meeting columnar epithelium, which lines cervix, at the os. Two poorly developed layers of muscle, external longitudinal and internal circular form middle layer. Outer covering is of connective tissue containing a rich plexus of blood vessels.

Uterus

Hollow muscular organ lying between bladder and rectum.

Size

Varies at different ages.

At puberty grows to $7.5 \times 5 \times 2.5$ cm with 1.25 cm thick muscular wall. Vast increase occurs during pregnancy with thinning of wall thickness to 0·5 cm. Post-parturition involution is rapid. Uterus almost back to pre-pregnancy size in one month. Post menopausal atrophy to half size.

Parts
Corpus or body forms main bulk. Upper rounded dome is fundus. Fallopian tubes attached below fundus at the cornuae (horns). Lower one third is cervix (neck).

Structure
Three layers; inner—endometrium, middle—myometrium, outer—perimetrium.

Endometrium. Thickness varies through menstrual cycle. Composed of connective stroma supporting tubular epithelial glands and their secretions.

Myometrium. Smooth muscle fibres closely interwoven and arranged so that contraction can squeeze shut the arterioles penetrating to endometrium.

Layers of muscle form internal circular layer, middle figure of eight pattern and outer longitudinal layer. Layers are poorly defined. Muscle thins out in lower third which becomes lower uterine segment during labour. Absent from cervix.

Perimetrium. Serous peritoneal layer continuous with broad ligament which extends laterally to pelvic walls and covers fallopian tubes and anterior surface of ovaries.

Cervix
Projects into vault of vagina. Opening into cavity of uterus centrally placed in cervix—external os. 2·3 cm within cervix cavity constricted to form internal os. Cervix composed of elastic tissue with very little muscle. Firm, rubbery consistency. Lined with mucous membrane secreting mucous which varies in consistency according to predominant hormone. Oestrogen phase of menstrual cycle mucous is thin watery and forms ferny pattern when dried on glass slide. Progesterone phase mucous becomes thick, tenacious and can be drawn out into long string.

Ligaments of uterus
Uterus supported by ligaments, thickened bands within peritoneum. Broad ligaments, round ligaments, utero sacral lig-

aments. Broad ligaments drape over uterus and tubes and extend laterally to pelvic walls dividing true pelvis into anterior portion containing bladder and posterior portion containing rectum. At level of cervix lowermost parts of broad ligament thickened to form transverse cervical ligaments (cardinal ligaments) which are main support for uterus. Damage or stretching of these ligaments predisposes to prolapse.

Round ligaments pass form cornuae in front and below junction of fallopian tubes. Pass forward through inguinal canals to disappear in tissues of labia majora.

Utero-sacral ligaments
Thickenings in pertoneum which pass from cervix to sacrum and prevent retroversion to some extend.

Fallopian tubes, ovaries, vessels, nerves, lymphatics form bulk of tissue between anterior and posterior surfaces of broad ligament. Ovaries not covered posteriorly—remain open into peritoneal space.

Fallopian tubes

Two muscular tubes 10 to 12 cm long attached to cornuae of uterus and communicating with its cavity.

Parts
Interstitial, 1·25 cm lies within thickness of uterine wall.

Isthmus, 1·25 cm narrowest part lies immediately outside wall of uterus.

Ampulla, 3·4 cm widest portion in which fertilization takes place.

Infundibulum, terminal trumpet-like part fringed by finger-like fimbriae in contact with ovary.

Structure
3 layers. Internal ciliated mucous membrane greatly convoluted and branched. Cilia help to create a current in the pervading mucous which helps to move ova to uterus.

Middle layer thick muscular tissue subdivided into outer longitudinal coat and inner circular coat. Peristaltic waves traverse tube aiding onward passage of ovum. Outer covering of peritoneum.

Ovaries

Oval, flattened glandular structures measuring 4 × 2 × 1·25 cm. Situated on posterior surface of broad ligament under curve of fallopian tube.

Parts

Cortex and medulla.

Cortex composed of layer of cubical cells which gives rise to structures from which ova derived—ovarian (Graafian) follicles. Medulla consists of stroma of spindle shaped cells supporting rich network of vessels and follicles. Follicles composed of layer of cells, granulosa cells, surrounding fluid filled space. Ovum surmounts hillock of granulosa cells, called the cumulus ovaricus, within the follicle space and is bathed in liquor folliculi. Under influence of FSH most advanced follicle undergoes maturation to produce fully developed ovum. At ovulation follicle ruptures discharging ovum with covering of zona pellucida and irregular layer of cells, the corona radiata.

Discharged follicle undergoes changes to become corpus luteum, which producess progesterone. If pregnancy occurs corpus luteum persists and grows for several months. If not, corpus luteum degenerates starting 2–3 days before onset of menstruation. Old corpora lutea remain as scars on ovary, corpora albicans. Development of corpus luteum controlled by LH.

Oestrogens produced by cells of developing follicles controlled by FSH.

Index

169

180   INDEX